"Like the author, I know as an athlete that my body functions better with exercise, yet as an internist and an oncologist, I know that many of my patients do not have a regular exercise program. I hope that *Active Against Cancer* can motivate some of my patients to use exercise to help themselves. I plan to make this book available to patients at my office."

– John Valentine, M.D., Mountainview Medical of
Central Vermont Medical Center, Berlin, Vermont

"I can't think of a more empowering way to fight cancer. Whether or not you are a seasoned athlete, this book should give you motivation and inspiration. Both professionally and personally, I have seen the benefits of activity over inactivity, on the mind and body, as presented in *Active Against Cancer*. The information is clear and sound. This book should be helpful reading for those diagnosed with cancer and those close to somebody fighting cancer."

– Donna Smyers, M.S., P.T.,
Six-time Ironman Age-group World Champion

"*Active Against Cancer* encourages you to get up, get out, and get some exercise. Author Nancy S. Brennan, a cancer survivor herself, speaks from her own experience and others' when she describes how exercising through cancer recovery can make you feel better physically, emotionally, and spiritually. Even when the going gets really tough, this book will motivate you to do some sort of daily workout, no matter how insignificant it may seem, because any workout is better than no workout. *Active Against Cancer* will inspire you to make exercise a habit you will look forward to, every day."

– Kate Carter, founder and former editor,
Vermont Sports magazine

"*Active Against Cancer* provides inspiration and practical advice for starting and continuing an exercise program during and after cancer treatment. For me, riding my bicycle to daily radiation therapy demonstrated to myself and to others that I–and not the treatments–was in control of my life and my health. I would recommend this encouraging book to help others who are facing cancer to be active in their own empowering ways."

– Barbara Pike, Nordic skier, cyclist,
cancer survivor, and adventurous outdoor athlete

"*Active Against Cancer* is both practical and inspirational, and it serves as a wonderful guide to move cancer survivors toward improved fitness. There is accumulating evidence that exercise is a key therapeutic component of cancer treatment. Exercise after initial cancer treatment may even help to prevent the recurrence of some cancers. Keeping active can help cancer survivors take some control during trying times."

– Kim Dittus, M.D., Ph.D.,
Oncologist / Hematologist, Burlington, Vermont

ACTIVE
AGAINST
CANCER

A Guide to

Improving Your Cancer Recovery

with Exercise

NANCY S. BRENNAN

Courage Mountain Press
861 Mountainview Drive
Duxbury VT 05676
www.couragemountainpress.com

First edition published 2011.

ISBN: 978-0-9834601-0-7

Acknowledgments:

Book design, publishing consulting, and cover design by Studio 6 Sense. More information at www.studio6sense.com.

Photographs of author on cover and back cover: ©Edward J. Brennan.

Editorial assistance: Kate Carter, Cotton Brook Publications, Waterbury, Vermont.

Thank you to the advance readers for review, comment, and encouragement.

Thank you to all the profiled cancer survivors for your time and generous sharing of your stories.

Thank you to friends, family, and professionals who helped me during my cancer challenge; thank you to all my sports' buddies; and to thank you to the cancer community for being the best club that I ever joined against my will.

This book is dedicated to my husband, Edward,
for sorbet, summits and our love.

And with love to my mother, Kay Smith, and
in loving memory of my father, Theodore Smith.

And to all who have a cancer challenge.

"If you want to get to the top of the hill,
you must go up it."

– Yankee Proverb

CONTENTS

INTRODUCTION

For the vast majority of people facing cancer, staying physically active during cancer treatment and beyond will provide significant benefits. This consensus of medical opinion is rippling through the institutions and organizations that care for cancer patients. The advice to exercise during cancer treatment will soon, if it is not already, be the standard.

What does this mean for you? It means that you should be physically active during your cancer recovery, if your limitations allow. This book will help you to plan your exercise activities appropriately and will help you succeed with them. The first chapter lays the groundwork for why exercise improves cancer recovery. Subsequent chapters discuss related medical programs, trends in patient care, and relevant medical considerations. Exercise plans, adjustments, and tips are described.

To help you imagine your success with exercise in cancer recovery, you will read, in detail, about ten cancer survivors who used exercise well and who healed successfully. The profiled cancer survivors received conventional medical care, such as surgery, chemotherapy, and radiation, which they primarily used to fight cancer. To that care, however, they added exercise.

The profiled active survivors had different backgrounds, levels of fitness, types of disease, types of activities that they enjoyed, and hardships that they faced during treatment. However, they shared one thing in common: a belief in the importance of exercise during cancer treatment. Stubbornly in some cases and matter-of-factly in others, they stayed committed to being physically active. Exercise, they thought, could make a difference and improve their recoveries. They were "active against cancer" and chose exercise over inactivity. By learning about their resolve, you may be able to deepen your own desire to use activity to help during your cancer challenge.

The first profile that I offer is mine. It's not any more or less important than the others, but I do know my story very well. You will have a good introduction to how one person was active against cancer, and, by the end of the profile, you will know me better.

MY PROFILE: ACTIVE AGAINST CANCER

Before my cancer diagnosis, I was seemingly healthy, fit and trim. In my middle age, I had a very active lifestyle with year-round participation in outdoor sports. Competing in Nordic ski racing since age thirty-four, I skied in a handful of citizen races each winter. My favorite event was the ski marathon, where I would ski thirty-two miles (50 km) in about four hours. In warmer months, I ran on hiking trails and hilly Vermont dirt roads. I swam, water-skied, hiked, and kept active with various running races. I competed in half-marathon races (13.1 miles) and I raced up mountain roads in several states. Doing year-round outdoor sports was a way of life. I treasured my fitness, my health, and my healthy lifestyle.

At age forty-seven, I met my life partner who is now my husband. Edward is an alpine skier, a hiker, a swimmer, and a water skier. He tutored me in making turns on alpine skis; I took him out on cross-country trails. We were happily making plans for the future when my cancer interrupted our lives.

For a few years, my stamina had felt unusually low. I had felt run down and burdened by a kind of constant fatigue. No matter how much I rested or how I tried to change my training, I felt sapped. I had cut back on racing but tried to keep up with exercise, despite undue fatigue.

Sometimes I worried that I had a big health problem. Ovarian cancer had crossed my mind more than once. Ovarian cancer deserves its reputation as being hard to diagnose. My symptoms included: bloating, urgency to urinate, feeling full after eating a small amount, two instances of severe pain in my abdomen, irregular menstrual cycles, and fatigue that would not relent. I also bruised easily and ate a lot more than usual without gaining weight. The problem was that I never added up all these things. One at a time, these symptoms did not set off alarms. By the time some of the last and more alarming symptoms arrived, I did add them up, but by then, my cancer was well established.

One evening, I felt a large unrecognized mass in my abdomen during my yoga class. I knew that I needed urgent medical help. Two days later, I went to the emergency room. After an abdominal scan, the doctor told me as gently as he could that I had a significant and worrisome mass. I immediately suspected it was my fear come true: ovarian cancer. The doctors would only know the answer after surgery.

Within a week, I had major surgery to remove the mass, which was, a malignant ovarian cancer tumor. My surgeon was a gynecological oncologist with much experience and expertise; I am forever grateful to him. Luckily, I had no evidence of metastatic disease. Because of the large tumor burden and other reasons, however, I was offered five months of rigorous chemotherapy with carboplatin and paclitaxel. I signed up without hesitation. Life before cancer had just ended. Life as a cancer patient had begun.

Cancer treatment was a very frightening and humbling time. Medically, things went extremely well, but that was the doctor's perspective, not necessarily mine at the time. During cancer treatment, the whole cancer ordeal felt surreal and full of unique challenges. No one finds receiving toxic chemicals in the blood stream to be routine the first time as a cancer patient.

I was so glad not to have metastatic cancer that I was able to keep my spirits up during treatment, but the months felt very long. The side effects felt like being pecked at by a hundred chickens. No one side effect, itself, was so bad, but in combination, they seemed overwhelming and frightening.

My oncologist commented that my overall fitness would help me heal faster and tolerate chemotherapy better. After surgery, I had been told that I could walk, if I wanted to, so I did. I began to walk, albeit slowly, on the second day after surgery. The next two days, I did laps in the hospital hallway, slow but steady. Walking with my fresh abdominal incision wasn't easy, but it felt better than lying helplessly in bed.

During the next five months of cancer treatment, I was advised that I could exercise but not to overdo it. Until the first six weeks post-surgery passed, I was to do no lifting, no swimming, and no high intensity aerobic activities. After that, it was up to me.

I walked outdoors for exercise, walking about twenty-five yards on my first day home. I worked up to being able to walk to the end of the 100-foot driveway. Then, I added more walking distance, incrementally, each time. I stayed on flat areas. I kept increasing the walking distance incrementally in the first six weeks of recovery. Some days I would walk two or three times for five to ten minutes each time. I walked slowly, but it was helping.

After six weeks, I swam. Going to the lake to swim felt like a luxuriously normal thing to do. Some days, I would merely pretend to be swimming. I would float on my back, look at the sky, and relax. Other days my freestyle or breaststroke had a little zip. I typically swam gently, slowly, with plenty of rest breaks. The distances and intensity were much less than in a normal year, but that was okay with me. Swimming was like a tonic to my battered spirits. I always felt lucky that I had my treatment in summer because it was warm and I could swim outdoors.

During my treatment, I just did whatever activity I could do each day, making sure that I tried to do something rather than do nothing. I didn't try to be fast or push hard. It was usually rewarding enough to just be moving, doing exercise that I found pleasant. I never tried to stress myself or be very ambitious. I tried to feel good.

I rarely used my fatigue as a reason to not go for a walk or a swim because I found I could adapt the pace to suit how I felt. Some days, climbing the stairs was tough. Other days, my fatigue was not as bad. Eventually, I could guess my hemoglobin numbers by how I felt climbing the stairs, a neat party trick that helped me feel more in control and less frightened by my fluctuating numbers.

My infusions were given every three weeks and the pattern of my roller-coaster energy levels eventually became familiar, though never routine. The day after chemotherapy, I would have some fresh energy and make good use of it. Then I would suffer for several days with various side effects. Next, my blood cell counts would sink lower in the middle of the second week, only to start to rise again before the next infusion. With each treatment session, I weakened and rebounded somewhat less well, but my numbers, to the doctor, were excellent. I was briefly anemic or neutropenic but never in dire straits.

I live on a hillside. When I go for a walk, I walk steeply downhill and then steeply uphill to return home. As my anemia worsened, my husband took to calling the uphill walk "my personal Everest." It felt like a high-altitude hike sometimes when my blood counts were low because I struggled to have enough oxygen reach my leg muscles. I would stop and rest, then continue on. Thinking of it as Mount Everest actually helped! I could imagine myself as a healthy person in thin air rather than a cancer patient with low hemoglobin. I could imagine using the same kind of conviction that mountaineers use to get to the top.

I did some especially fun activities during chemotherapy. Once, more than halfway into five months of treatments, I hiked to the top of my favorite local mountain. My husband and I had planned a short hike on the trail. When I didn't feel like quitting, we just kept going. After resting often and walking slowly—not to mention receiving a free sandwich from a stranger—I made it to the summit. Ordinarily, the hike to the summit would take me less than two hours. This time, it took me about four hours to reach the top. I was bald, tired, grateful, and ecstatic. I felt, on the summit, that I was winning and cancer was losing. (The cover of this book shows me on same summit on my forty-ninth birthday, six weeks after treatment ended.)

The other especially fun treat was water-skiing, which was ordinarily a common summertime activity for me. During chemotherapy, I did my slalom water skiing a few times a month, overlapping with the times when I felt best. I skied with less vigor and more caution than usual, but water skiing was joyous. It made me feel strong and victorious over cancer, even if only symbolically. I'm sure I enjoyed a hit of endorphins, as well.

My chemotherapy was bringing down my tumor marker count in excellent fashion, so the results of treatment were a significant help to my morale. (In my cancer type, tumor marker counts reveal active disease. Having their numbers go down is ideal.) My side effects were routine, as these things go. They sometimes seemed awful to me, but they were not medically worrisome. Perhaps most troubling to me was that I had some problems with peripheral neuropathy in my feet. I had some tingling, pain, and mild numb-like symptoms that were more annoying than anything else. I had a timely, expert neurology consult that helped me to be optimistic about the neuropathy's likelihood of resolving after treatment. The assessment showed that my damage was actually minor so far. I couldn't damage my nerves by walking, so I just made sure that I was careful not to trip.

During my treatment, my modified sports activities didn't make me more tired. Walking or swimming each gave me a gentle boost in energy right away, so I was always up for some activity. I had insomnia very badly. Doing some activity each day perhaps helped me sleep better than I would have without it.

I definitely ate better because of exercise, which worked to quell my mild chemo-related nausea and to stimulate my appetite. With my particular cancer and treatment, being able to keep appropriate weight on during treatment is an excellent sign. I couldn't gain weight, but I didn't lose more. Exercise helped me to stay relatively fit and strong. Being strong enough to water-ski was a good test. I didn't worry about losing some cardiovascular fitness; I knew it could come back.

I have just as many good memories from my chemotherapy summer as I do from some other summers—and almost all of them involve being active outdoors and having fun with sports or walking. Being active helped me keep part of my identity intact.

It helped me feel strong and determined. Being active made it easier to imagine that I would recover my full health. I suffered in many ways during chemotherapy, but I'm so glad that I gave myself the gift of being active throughout the ordeal.

WHY I WROTE THIS BOOK

One year after my treatment ended, I read Dr. David Servan-Shreiber's book, *Anticancer, A New Way of Life*. Dr. Servan-Schreiber is an eloquent writer, a medical doctor, and a long-term brain cancer survivor. He helped to popularize the word "anti-cancer," which he used to describe those non-medical self-care choices that work against cancer. Anticancer self-care choices can include strategic choices about diet, rest, and exercise.

Reading *Anticancer*, I learned about how cancer's progress could be defeated on the biochemical level by the changes that take place when a person exercises. On the cellular level, cancer thrives in an inflammatory environment. By being anti-inflammatory, if you will, exercise is anticancer. This is just one example of why exercise helps fight cancer. More details are described in the next chapter. In total, exercise is an anticancer activity as Dr. Servan-Schreiber describes it.

After reading his book, I started to think about how much value my physical activities might have had in actually fighting my cancer. I was extremely glad that I had chosen to stay active during cancer treatment. After reading *Anticancer*, I felt even more empowered against the threat of recurrence. When I went out the door to walk, run or hike, after reading his book, I imagined that I was getting farther from the cancer threat with each step. What a powerful motivator. What if, during my treatment, I had fully appreciated how valuable exercise was in helping my body heal from cancer? What extra self-empowerment and mental relief could I have experienced?

I wrote this book so that you can appreciate the value of being active in your cancer recovery. You can be active against cancer every time you get some exercise. I believe that being active can be fun and a real blessing to your life. To keep it simple for you, I have written a very practical guide with exercise programs that you can do yourself. You can use this book if your treating hospital does not have a therapeutic exercise program tailored for you to use. You can succeed with a home-based, independent program of your own or you can combine it with community resources at your fitness center. Walking and other common sports activities, as well as other favorite activities that provide exercise, form the basis of the exercise plans. No matter what sports you like, you should be able to adapt these plans to work for you.

For the exercise plans, I have followed the guidelines established by the American College of Sports Medicine, the American Cancer Society, and other related organizations. This book can help you to get started safely. You will read about tips for success and I can help you find a pattern of exercise or activity that you can enjoy. I can help you know how to adjust your exercise levels during treatment. Topics related to side effects are discussed, along with precautions and contraindications.

Please check with your medical caregivers before beginning any exercise program. That is not an empty, merely routine disclaimer. If you are in cancer treatment or recovery, no advice in this book should be substituted for individualized medical care from professionals who know your health history and your current health status in detail. It isn't possible for an author to know which cancer you struggle against, nor to know what stage of disease, what prognosis, what side effects, or type of treatment you are receiving. Use this book for the basis of a discussion with your doctor and caregivers. You are responsible for seeking appropriate advice from your own medical team.

Lastly, I have a prejudice to share when it comes to sports, fitness, and physical activities. I believe that being active can be fun. Please try to keep an element of fun-loving spirit in your approach to activity. Your body is not a machine. While you are active during your cancer recovery, I hope you can envision exercise as valuable medicine, but it is also much more than medicine. Being active can soothe your soul.

You can appreciate the immeasurable goodness of a walk in the spring air, a bike ride with cancer survivors, or a Tai Chi class on a lakeshore. Physical activity can provide you with comfort, calm and renewal, or with determination, grit and strength. Some days you may just need to get your exercise done, but on other days, your activity choice can make you happy while it also helps you to have a better cancer recovery.

CANCER AS THE UNINVITED HOUSEGUEST

When cancer comes into your life, it often barges in like an uninvited, unruly, self-centered houseguest. You must drop everything and deal with whatever demands cancer makes. Nothing else is as important. Cancer is a major bully. Facing cancer will become your top priority. Cancer can, and usually does, turn your daily life upside down.

However, there may come a time, after cancer has been living in your house a while, when some of its demands start to be predictable and almost bearable. Then you may find that you can sneak some time away from cancer. You can slip out the back door while it's napping and go do something of your own choosing.

When you find those free hours, you can take care of yourself by doing some pleasurable physical activities that help to restore your calm, build your strength, reinforce your courage, and, ultimately, help your good cells kick out those unwanted, unruly cancer cells. One day, when you get back to your home from an especially rewarding adventure, you may discover that your uninvited guest, cancer, has packed up and left you for good. I hope that you will have such a day soon.

I wish you many happy steps on your trail back to health and many cancer-free years.

With peace,
Nancy

CHAPTER ONE

WHY BEING ACTIVE IMPROVES CANCER RECOVERY

Cancer is not one disease. Cancer is comprised of many diseases that have in common the uncontrolled reproduction of cancer cells. These cancer cells become harmful to your body in a variety of ways, depending on the cancer type and its progression. Frequently, cancer cells create tumors that create difficulties in the functioning of their own or nearby organs or body parts. The primary tumor can cause life-threatening damage, or it may also send cancer cells into the bloodstream, which may cause the cancer to spread.

The medical term for cancer spreading beyond the initial site is "metastasizing," as you probably know. If a tumor metastasizes, then cancer cells are sent to other parts of the body where they may start new tumors or uncontrolled growth. The metastatic cancer often becomes dangerous to your health, in itself, even if the primary tumor has been removed or controlled with chemotherapy.

What is the cause of cancer cells' uncontrolled reproduction of themselves? Here is a simple, yet accurate, way to understand this phenomenon more deeply. As you may recall from high school biology class, your entire body is made up of cells. The cells in your body become distinct from one another by having special functions. Biologists call this "differentiation." That word may sound imposing, but all it means is that cells have different roles to play: A cell on the outer layer of your skin is different from a cell inside your muscle fiber, which is different from a hair cell or a fingernail cell and so on. The cells are differentiated, and to be so, they are expressing different parts of the genetic code in a way that restricts their roles to the role appropriate to that part of the body.

Each type of cell in your body has a pattern of how often it reproduces, how it functions, how it decides how long to last, and when to die off naturally. The process of dying off, as a cell, is another fancy word, "apoptosis." Generally, the fastest reproducing cells in the human body are these: hair cells, skin cells, the cells lining your digestive tract, and the blood cells being produced in your bone marrow. These cells serve the body best by undergoing relatively frequent apoptosis.Those of you who have had certain types of chemotherapy may notice that these fast-reproducing cells are the same ones that your chemotherapy damaged, along with the cancer cells. This idea gives us a clue about a feature of most, not all, cancer cells: They reproduce quickly. They are nearly constantly trying to make copies of themselves. Most chemotherapy works by trying to kill all fast-growing cells in your body, a group that includes most cancer cells. Incidentally—and unfortunately—the chemotherapy that is trying to eliminate cancer cells may kill your hair cells, skin cells, and the lining of your digestive tract cells, as well as interfere with blood production in your bones.

Those incidental problems are the bane of the chemotherapy patient, although advances in chemotherapy agents and dosing have resulted in improvements over the years. However, there is a limit to how much chemotherapy a patient can tolerate if all the body's fast-growing cells are damaged. Future chemotherapeutic agents may avoid these side effects by exploiting the differences between cancer cells and normal cells more precisely. Instead of killing all the fast-reproducing cells, the new agents may be able to target cancer cells directly. Research continues to search for these more tolerable approaches to chemotherapy.

Generally, we might ask ourselves: "Why are cancer cells doing something destructive to our bodies?" Cancer cells have had their genetic material altered so that they reproduce exact copies of themselves over and over again. The healthy body does not need these cells. The cells of some tumors also become non-differentiated, which means that they are not restricted to a specific appropriate cell function. Non-differentiated cells no longer resemble cells of the original type of cell at all. They are cells without a functional role, simply reproducing themselves rapidly. These cancer cells have terrible potential to overwhelm the health of nearby organs, enter blood vessels and the lymph system, spread copies of themselves to distant organs and begin new tumors, and, ultimately, exact a toll on a body's health. Some cancers are categorized as more aggressive because of the presence of non-differentiated cells that are highly able to cause havoc.

PRO-CANCER CONDITIONS IN THE BODY

Cancer cells create certain conditions as their numbers grow. They change the local cellular environment by changing the biochemistry. Furthermore, cancer cells favor certain biochemical conditions in order to reproduce. Sometimes cancer cells are overwhelmed by the immune system response of the body and they die. Other times, the cancer cells' growth is encouraged by conditions that they favor. Conditions of the body that favor cancer growth can include:

1. Inflammation at the cellular level;
2. Greater levels of insulin or insulin-like growth factor;
3. Poorly oxygenated blood;
4. Too much cortisol, a natural stress hormone;
5. Excessive levels of sex hormones, such as estrogen or testosterone;

6. Obesity;

7. A weakened immune system;

8. And poor nutritional intake, favoring excessive fat production and high blood sugar levels.

There is good news, however. The opposite of these conditions can be called "anticancer conditions." Anticancer conditions are bad for the continued uncontrolled reproduction of cancer cells. In fact, this is extremely good news because it means that there are many simple ways to make your body less hospitable to cancer cells. Medical science can actually show us how to help our bodies create anticancer conditions that are the opposite of the list above. Let's look at the opposite of the previous list, briefly.

ANTICANCER CONDITIONS IN THE BODY

1. Anti-inflammatory cellular environment;

2. Moderate levels of insulin and insulin-like growth factor;

3. Well-oxygenated blood;

4. Moderate levels of cortisol;

5. Moderate levels of sex hormones;

6. Appropriate body-weight;

7. A strong immune system;

8. Good or optimum nutritional intake.

Look carefully at that list. If you eat well and not too much, and if you get a good volume of exercise, you can actively promote anticancer conditions in the cellular environment of your body. Read that again: If you eat well and not too much, and if you get a good volume of exercise, you can actively promote anticancer conditions in the cellular environment of your body.

FIVE ANTICANCER EFFECTS OF EXERCISE

The anticancer benefits of frequent moderate exercise are described in medical detail in the following list. Exercise, in moderation, helps to create the desirable anticancer conditions in your body at a cellular level, thereby helping you fight cancer with exercise.

1. Exercise can reduce levels of cellular inflammation by lowering blood sugar levels, reducing insulin and insulin-like growth factor.

2. Exercise provides a boost to your immune system.

3. Exercise lowers your stress levels and brings stress hormones to a beneficial level.

4. Exercise can regulate important sex hormones such as estrogen and testosterone.

5. Exercise keeps your body fat low, your weight appropriate, and improves your body composition (the mixture of fat and muscle).

Let's look at each of these topics in more detail in the following sections.

Exercise Can Reduce Cellular Inflammation

Frequent, moderate exercise can reduce inflammation at the cellular level. Cancer "likes" inflammation. Tumor activity can both increase inflammation and be enhanced by the inflammation. That's not what you want! You want an anti-inflammatory cellular environment. A good anticancer goal is to reduce inflammation in the body through dietary choices and physical activity.

How does exercise in moderation reduce inflammation? It lowers your blood sugar and helps to keep your circulating insulin at an optimum level. This process reduces inflammation. By controlling the levels of insulin and insulin-like growth factor (IGF), which is a similar chemical, exercise makes a cellular environment that is less conducive to cancer growth.

Here's an example of what that might mean for you. Let's say that you ate six donuts at one sitting. I'm not saying you would do that, but if you ate six donuts, your insulin level would rise. In response to the sugars and foods consumed, insulin is released from your pancreas. The rising insulin level helps the body reduce the amount of sugar circulating in the blood and get your blood sugar back into a normal range as quickly as possible. If you ate six donuts every hour all day, you would raise your blood sugar frequently, and then your pancreas, if healthy, would release spiking amounts of insulin in an attempt to lower your blood sugar. You would, in total, have more insulin in your blood than is optimum.

Cancer cells behave as if insulin is a growth factor for them, and by this, I mean that insulin makes cancer cells grow. Insulin creates, on the level of biochemistry, a very friendly environment for cancer cells. Excess insulin causes inflammation; inflammation, in the cellular environment, is pro-cancer and, in short, is bad for your health. Insulin-like growth factor also contributes to the undesired inflammatory conditions.

You want to have the opposite of increasing cellular inflammation. You want a fairly even blood sugar level and optimal lower levels of circulating insulin and IGF. Exercise, in moderate amounts, helps you accomplish this. Exercise directly and immediately lowers your insulin level and evens out blood sugar regulation. Moderate, frequent exercise regulates your blood sugar, helps keep insulin levels optimal, and helps create a cellular environment that is not inflammatory. Additionally, with a healthy amount of exercise, you reduce your likelihood of contracting diabetes, a disease that increases cellular inflammation.

Exercise is not the only way to reduce inflammation. Dietary choices, as we have seen, are important. Certain foods and spices like turmeric, which is in many curries, reduce inflammation. A glass of wine can reduce inflammation. Recently, aspirin has been recognized as having anticancer effects in terms of colon cancer and perhaps others. Is this because aspirin is anti-inflammatory? Perhaps. More understanding of the value of anti-inflammatory agents will come to light in the future because this area of research is quite promising and active right now.

Exercise Provides a Boost to Your Immune System

The immune system of the human body is both enormously complex and fascinating, but exploring its details is far beyond the scope of this book. However, it is well known that the immune system benefits from regular, moderate exercise.

Most of us know that we should stay in bed and rest if we have a horrible case of the flu, a fever, or other severe illness. When you have a head-cold, if you take a short walk of 5 to 10 minutes, the activity boosts your immune system and helps you heal faster. Isn't that great? Spending some time with your heart rate raised by exertion and your muscles moving immediately provides a boost to your immune system. By nature, we are animals who benefit from moving.

Exercise promotes, among other things, an increase in the number of natural killer cells, which are white blood cell components of the immune system. The natural killer cells of the immune system are capable of killing cancer cells. (Yes, that's really what they're called: natural killer cells.) By using exercise to help boost your production of natural killer cells, you are helping your immune system fight cancer more effectively.

Certainly, strengthening the immune system is more complex than increasing just the natural killer cells, but for me, that one part of the picture is persuasive. Simply knowing that activity helps my immune system makes me want to be active during cancer recovery. It's difficult to convey how important optimal immune system function is to your health. Let's say: extraordinarily.

Exercise Lowers Your Stress and Moderates Cortisol Level

As is the case for many chemicals in the body, there is an optimal level for your stress hormones. Cortisol is an important stress hormone. Most people who have a cancer health crisis will have a rise in their cortisol levels, caused by increased stress levels.

Stress levels rise because you may have significant pain, intense fears, disturbed routines, sleep loss, many extra concerns, and stressful medical visits, among other things. We each experience cancer differently, but I think we can agree that a cancer diagnosis is stressful.

Cortisol as a short-term response to an injury, for example, acts to reduce inflammation. However, when stress levels are high for the long term, the increased levels of cortisol are immuno-suppressing, that is, they reduce your immune system function. High levels of cortisol over a long period are cancer-friendly. Fortunately, exercise can reduce both your stress level and your associated cortisol level.

In times of high stress, have you ever gone for a short walk with a friend and felt much better about your situation afterwards? Have you gone for a hike all tense and ended up all relaxed and feeling more optimistic? Exercise lowers your cortisol level and helps you feel less stressed. At the same time that you are relaxing better, you are lowering your cortisol level to a more optimal level. Don't worry if you haven't always found exercising to be relaxing: You can learn to. I'll be providing some tips to help you.

Exercise Helps Regulate Sex Hormones

Hormones and hormone regulation are also complex, biochemi-cally. It is well agreed upon that moderate, frequent exercise helps to regulate sex hormones such as estrogen and testos-terone. Exercise helps your body control these hormones so that they can reach optimal levels. In contrast, excessive amounts of sex hormones can contribute to cancers, including breast cancer, gynecological cancers or testicular cancer. Exercise can help keep their levels at their best.

In addition, some sex hormones, especially estrone, a form of estrogen, are produced in fat tissue. If you have excessive amounts of body fat, you have higher levels of estrogen, gener-ally. Exercise can help you keep body fat levels low and keep your sex hormone levels in the ideal range.

Exercise Keeps Your Body Fat Low

It's obvious to most of us that exercise helps you keep your body fat low. Why does a lower body fat volume help against cancer? There are several reasons, one of which I have just mentioned. Body fat produces some estrogen, and too much estrogen is a burden. In addition, body fat is a storage area for toxic chemicals that may be carcinogenic. Less fat means less toxic burden for the body.

There may also be contributions to cellular inflammation simply from excess fat storage. Higher body fat can be related to food choices that promote diabetes development, which produces higher insulin levels, which in turn promote cancer.

Although the effects of excessive body fat are somewhat complex, it's true that having too much body fat is connected to a variety of negative effects on health. These negative effects include higher risk of getting breast or other cancers and higher risk of cancer mortality in breast, colorectal, and other cancers. Lower body fat is good for your cancer-related health.

Finally, it is easier to do many types of exercise if you are weight-appropriate. Exercise can help you lose weight, and being trimmer can help you exercise more easily. Exercising can provide all the benefits described above and more. Sometimes the only difficulty is getting started on the right exercise program. Keep reading!

FUNCTIONAL ANTICANCER BENEFITS OF EXERCISE

Along with important cellular processes and biochemical realities, exercise also provides benefits to your overall health in ways that are more easily understandable and no less important. During a cancer challenge, your sense of your own vitality and well-being will greatly affect your self-care choices such as those choices about eating well, getting enough sleep, staying involved in activity, and feeling good despite the burdens of illness.

How can exercise specifically affect your health in ways that help your body to fight cancer? Here is our second set of reasons to exercise. I call them the functional reasons because they emphasize ways that exercise helps you function better during cancer treatment. They are the results of exercise that you, yourself, can feel and appreciate. They reflect many of the underlying biological and biochemical processes that were just described, but this next list will seem less like science-class material than the preceding section.

Here are the functional reasons why exercise helps you fight cancer.

1. Exercise improves perceived energy levels and sense of well-being.

2. Exercise helps you sleep well and receive the benefits of sleep.

3. Exercise supports healthy eating habits, improves digestive prowess, and helps control appetite naturally.

4. Exercise lifts mood, promotes healthy self-care choices, and guards against depression.

5. Exercise increases fitness and strength, which help the body in times of illness.

Most of these claims have been studied, and fortunately, most of the claims also match our own experiences. They pass for common sense, which is very good.

Exercise Improves Energy Level and Sense of Well-being

For most people, having cancer is an ordeal that causes a lot of stress. Feelings of fear, anxiety, and heightened vulnerability are common. (If you have had cancer, I'm sure I don't need to point this out to you.) In order to cope with the demands of cancer treatment, you will need a lot of emotional, mental, and physical energy. It takes stamina, both mentally and physically, to cope with the challenges of cancer in your life. Having extra energy would be ideal.

However, many patients receive necessary cancer treatments that cause physical fatigue. The fatigue comes from changes in blood composition, such as anemia or low white blood cell counts. Fatigue can also come from periods of forced inactivity such as may occur after a surgery, during times of feeling unwell, or because of treatment side effects. A low energy level from any of these causes tends to not be relieved by rest or more sleep.

Exercise has been shown to provide both short-term and long-term relief from the type of fatigue of cancer patients in treatment experience. Frequent, moderate exercise can lead to a lessening of fatigue during cancer treatment and also after treatment has ended. A peer-reviewed medical study confirmed this while studying breast cancer patients, leading more physicians to be interested in promoting exercise for their patients.

A great side effect of exercise is that you have more energy. If I begin exercising daily after a lay-off, I notice immediately that my energy levels go up, assuming that I don't over-do it. People who don't exercise are often surprised at this claim, but think of some people who are athletic. Do they seem to have a lot of energy? Generally, yes. Athletes tend to have more stamina and more energy than those who are more sedentary.

If you are going through cancer treatment, don't you want more stamina, more energy, and an uptick in your sense of your own well-being? Exercise can provide just that on a daily basis, as well as make a difference cumulatively over the long-term, even after treatment ends.

It is beyond the scope of this book to get into why, physiologically, exercise reduces fatigue and improves energy levels. Reasons include: raising the rate of blood circulation, strengthening the heart muscle, sweating out toxins, and improving digestion. All of these things probably contribute to making you feel better.

Some medical researchers are also looking into how hemoglobin levels may be raised by exercise. (Low hemoglobin levels cause anemia, which is correlated with fatigue.) Although the research is not complete on this topic, it is logical that moderate exercise would help your bone marrow boost production of blood cells.

Exercise Helps You Sleep Well and Receive Sleep's Benefits

Sleep is a treasured part of good health. During sleep, you receive many physiological benefits, including immune system benefits, reduction in stress, a rebalancing of chemicals that affect mood, and rest for muscles. In short, sleep is a time of healing for the body. With poor sleep, your health can suffer. Also, a bad night's sleep can lead to a poor mood, a feeling of tiredness, and a feeling of un-wellness. None of those effects are popular!

Cancer patients are not the world's best sleepers. We may have digestive problems that bother us at night. We may take certain drugs, such as corticosteroids, that make us feel alert. We may wake-up in the night from other side effects of our treatments. Some women in cancer treatment may be in sudden menopause after removal of ovaries, because of chemotherapy's overall burdens, or because of hormone-blocking medication. Menopause can make sleep a challenge. Fear, a high stress level, or disruptions in routine may disrupt our sleeping patterns. Whatever has chipped away at our sleep, we may suffer a bit.

With sleep loss often comes lowered cognitive function, or as some call it, "brain mush," which is the subjective feeling of not being sharp mentally. You probably know what it's like to be tired and fuzzy-headed. Good sleep, naturally, is valuable and courted. Frequent, regular exercise can help you sleep better. Exercise, by improving your sleep quality, can help your mood, your fatigue, your stress level, and your sense of feeling better.

Some active healthy people might relish pushing themselves to the point of exhaustion with sports, then sleeping deeply afterwards. However, during active cancer treatment, it is not medically advisable to get so tired from exercise that you are exhausted. You don't want to exert yourself so much that you are taxing your body's reserves during a time when you are in treatment. Your sleep quality can benefit from non-exhausting regular exercise, instead.

Exercise Supports Healthy Eating and Improves Digestion

If you exercise often enough, you will probably find that you are more apt to choose healthy foods, digest your food in a way that feels better, and have better success with controlling your appetite. Exercise raises your metabolism, which partly explains how it helps your digestion. You will find that exercise stimulates your digestive processes so that you process your food more quickly than in the absence of exercise. This stimulation helps in many ways, not least of all when you are fighting the constipation that comes with some chemotherapy.

Psychologically, you may want to protect your investment in exercise by making more healthy food choices and not overeating. If you eat lousy food, you will not feel as good when you exercise as if you eat healthy food. It doesn't take most people very long to figure that out. Eating well becomes very rewarding, because good fuel means having good energy.

Exercise can also help regulate your blood sugar levels, making you less prone to being overly hungry, chomping on sweets to get by, and making you more likely to eat appropriately. Snacking on a food with protein and fat, such as almonds, during an hour or more of exercise can help your energy levels.

Many people recognize that eating well during cancer recovery can be an important way to help their own healthfulness. Why not use exercise to help you to naturally crave better foods in the right portion sizes? Chemotherapy can harm the lining of the digestive tract and contribute to side effects like constipation, nausea, or vomiting. Anything that can improve digestion is welcome.

Happily, exercise can help reduce nausea immediately. After your stomach calms, you may feel better and want to eat the food that your body needs. Do try to use a short walk to control mild, but not severe, nausea. With the nausea lifted, you'll be more likely to eat a small amount, which will further help reduce your nausea and improve your energy.

Exercise Lifts Mood and Promotes Healthy Self-care

Exercise can enhance your sense of your own well-being. Physical activity can lift your mood. Studies consistently show that exercise is effective in treating mild to moderate depression. If you have achieved a better mood and avoided depression, you are more likely to make wise decisions in terms of self-care.

Let's imagine a fictional cancer patient called Alison. She is starting to be overwhelmed by depression-causing thoughts: "I can't handle this cancer" or "I'm not handling my treatment well." "I don't know if I can go on like this," she might think.

Then, one day her friend, Sunny, comes over and they decide to go for a short walk. By the end of the activity, Alison's mood has lifted. As the pair walked, Alison felt her muscles' strength and, despite being tired, she made contact with her sense of being a strong person. As she did, Alison felt more like herself and happier.

At the end of the walk and their conversation, Alison had resolved to follow-up on some ideas for better nutrition and to call the oncology nurse with a question about her digestive issues. She no longer is dwelling on feeling helpless or overwhelmed. Sunny volunteers to come by for a walk again next week, but Alison also resolves to go on a walk every day that she can, even if only for 15 minutes.

Over the next month, Alison feels more emotionally strong. Her depressive thoughts are much less frequent and she has more days when she thinks she can handle her health challenges. In fact, in some ways, Alison notices that, emotionally, with routine exercise, she is starting to be more upbeat than she has been in a long time. She sees the light at the end of the cancer tunnel.

What helped Alison? Getting moving helped her feel better. Maybe her serotonin levels went up, which exercise tends to do. Having better serotonin levels makes her feel better. Maybe she enjoyed some natural endorphins from exercise, which helped her mood. Maybe she slept better, over a few weeks, and being rested then helped her avoid depression. Importantly, exercise can help improve your mood in the short term and over the longer term.

Exercise Increases Fitness and Strength

Medical studies show that being fit is an advantage when recovering from surgery or a severe illness. Having low body fat, a good amount of lean muscle, excellent liver function, and a strong heart and circulatory system can benefit you when you have a health challenge. Doctors notice that people who are strong and fit, at any age, rebound better from physical challenges like surgery or illness.

Being active, that is, physically active, against cancer is a smart strategy for all the reasons that we have discussed in this chapter. There are so many reasons to exercise as you go through cancer treatment or recover from cancer. Let's turn to how medical doctors are integrating the research about exercise into recommendations and programs for cancer survivors.

CHAPTER TWO

MEDICAL ADVICE TO CANCER PATIENTS: BE ACTIVE

Medical opinion about activity during cancer treatment has evolved over time. Patients who experienced chemotherapy and radiation several decades ago often suffered more debilitating side effects than patients do today. Hospitalizations and life-threatening complications were possible for many patients. Advising very sick cancer patients to exercise in between episodes of high fever, severe nausea, low immune function, and debilitating weakness would have been unthinkable for physicians. Often, patients with only moderate side effects were simply told to rest or take it easy in order to get through treatment. The goals of treatment were to eradicate cancer and for the patient to survive the treatment.

Now, with advances in chemotherapy regimens, more targeted types of radiation therapy, and more advanced drugs to reduce side effects, such as nausea and anemia, many people in cancer treatment can reasonably be told to exercise.

In fact, advising cancer patients to be physically active during cancer treatment, within some limits, experts believe, is the medically sound advice that doctors should be giving. "Avoid inactivity" is the new standard guidance for patients who are recovering from cancer. This advice is endorsed by cancer experts, medical doctors, and esteemed cancer-related organizations. The advice to be active has a growing body of medical research behind it, as well as a groundswell of exercise programs for people in cancer recovery. Let's look at the recognition of the value of physical activity during cancer recovery in more detail.

EXERCISE GUIDELINES FOR CANCER SURVIVORS

In June 2010, the keynote speaker at the American Society of Clinical Oncology's annual meeting was Kathryn Schmitz, Ph.D., M.P.H., an associate professor of epidemiology (the study of disease) and biostatistics, and a member of the Abramson Cancer Center at the University of Pennsylvania School of Medicine. As the lead author of the report named *American College of Sports Medicine's Roundtable on Exercise Guidelines for Cancer Survivors* (hereafter, *Exercise Guidelines for Cancer Survivors*), Dr. Schmitz told the attending oncologists (cancer-treating doctors) that cancer patients should be active during cancer treatment, if possible.

Dr. Schmitz told the assemblage of oncologists: "The risk for cancer patients of 'doing nothing' is so great that it's best to just get [them] started with something." Summarizing the advice that the doctors should give directly to patients, Dr. Schmitz said, "The idea that you [cancer patients] should be staying put and resting is ultimately doing more harm than good."

The *Exercise Guidelines for Cancer Survivors* was published just prior to Dr. Schmitz' speech at the oncology conference in June 2010. Encompassing the review of 140 relevant medical and scientific studies, Dr. Schmitz and twelve highly credentialed colleagues from academia and medicine authored the guidelines after lengthy study. In their findings, they concluded: "Exercise is safe during and after cancer treatments and [it] results in improvements in physical functioning, quality of life, and cancer-related fatigue in several cancer survivor groups." Dr. Schmitz emphasized the two-word summary of advice that cancer patients should receive: "Avoid inactivity." In other words: get moving; be active; exercise.

The *Exercise Guidelines for Cancer Survivors* advised that cancer patients, after making any medically necessary adjustments, follow the same optimal exercise guidelines that healthy people follow. Cancer patients should be encouraged to get 30 minutes of exercise five days per week, above their usual daily activities, for a total of 150 minutes each week of moderate-intensity exercise. Strength training should be performed two or three times per week, addressing major muscle groups. Flexibility work should also be included. The *Exercise Guideline for Cancer Survivors'* authors emphasized that even during difficult cancer treatment or when active disease was present, cancer patients should still be encouraged to do appropriate exercise.

The *Exercise Guidelines for Cancer Survivors* recommendations for cancer patients are based on the ACSM's own 2008 exercise guidelines for all people. Just as exercise is good for anyone's health, it is good for the health of cancer patients. In addition, the guidelines also were influenced by the recommendations of the American Heart Association, the American Cancer Society, and the 2008 U.S. Department of Health and Human Services in their *Physical Activities for Americans Report*. There is, as a result of this collaboration, a thoughtful consensus on what cancer patients should do for exercise. The general recommendation is that during cancer treatment, patients should be "as physically active as their abilities and conditions allow." As simple as that may sound, it is also profound and important advice.

Let's look at the ACSM's *Exercise Guidelines For Cancer Survivors* in more detail. The report lists eight goals of the "exercise prescription." The goals of exercise for cancer recovery are:

1. Improving and restoring physical function, aerobic capacity, strength and flexibility.

2. Improving a patient's body self-image and quality of life.

3. Improving the ratio of strength to weight, called "body composition."

4. Improving cardiovascular and lung function, hormone systems function, muscle function, cognition (thinking skills), and psychosocial outcomes.

5. Potentially, to reduce or delay recurrence or a second primary cancer.

6. Improving one's coping with anxiety about recurrence or future cancer treatment.

7. Reducing or preventing negative long-term effects of cancer treatment, such as from chemotherapy or radiation.

8. Improving one's ability to mentally or physically withstand current or possibly future cancer treatments.

Best of all, there is agreement that the value of exercise is valid across most cancer diagnoses or treatments.

Take note of the fifth reason to exercise on this list: "Potentially, to reduce or delay recurrence or a second primary cancer." Although I have re-worded the rest of the above list, I have quoted that statement's exact wording because it is so important to see in its entirety. The number of studies that point to exercise as reducing or delaying recurrence or other cancer are limited, but the experts on the panel agreed on the validity of the claim that exercise might potentially help in this very significant regard.

Although more research is underway addressing this issue, if you are a cancer survivor, you can include in your personal motivation to exercise the ACSM panel's conclusion that exercise may help some cancer patients to live longer and be cancer-free longer. No one knows how statistics will apply to you individually, but if you are looking for motivation and hope, please remember that exercise is recognized as beneficial to your chances of survival. "There is increasing evidence that exercise not only benefits patients from the perspective of their well-being, it also appears to have an effect on reducing cancer recurrence rates and improving survival," said medical oncologist Danny Sims, M.D.

The well-known authority, the American Cancer Society, agrees that exercise is appropriate in cancer recovery. On their 2010 website, the American Cancer Society wrote that doctors telling patients to "rest and reduce their physical activity" was out-of-date advice. "Newer research has shown that exercise is not only safe and possible during cancer treatment, but it can improve physical functioning and quality of life." In recognizing that many cancer care teams are already making the switch to telling their patients to be as "physically active as possible during cancer treatment," the American Cancer Society weighed in with their opinion. "Regular exercise is an effective way to counteract the negative effects of inactivity in chronic illness," their website stated. Without a hint of controversy, the major cancer non-profit organization in the United States agrees that physical activity benefits cancer recovery.

The opinion of the National Cancer Institute is similarly in favor of physical activity in the fight against cancer. In their publicly available guidelines published on their website in 2010, they presented the case for exercising during cancer recovery. They also included detailed summaries about completed relevant medical studies on the topic. They wrote: "There is strong evidence that physical activity is associated with reduced risk of cancers of the colon and breast. Several studies have also reported links between physical activity and reduced risk of endometrial, lung and prostate cancers. Current National Cancer Institute studies are exploring the role of physical activity in cancer survivorship and quality of life, cancer risk, and the needs of populations at increased risk."

CANCER CENTERS AND HOSPITALS PROMOTE BEING ACTIVE

In the future, an increasing number cancer programs at hospitals may support patients in their exercise programs similarly to how their cardiac rehabilitation programs include exercise. As Kim Dittus, M.D., Ph.D., a medical oncologist and researcher in the field of exercise and cancer, said at the Breast Cancer Conference in Stowe, Vermont, in October 2010, "We're not to the point of [being like] cardiac rehab, but hopefully we will be getting there." Citing the ACSM's comprehensive *Exercise Guidelines for Cancer Survivors*, Dr. Dittus said: "Exercise is a prescription that should be given. There's a lot of research in support of exercise."

In fact, some major medical centers are already supporting cancer patients with hospital-based exercise programs. At the Norris Cotton Cancer Center's program for breast cancer survivors at Dartmouth-Hitchcock Medical Center in Lebanon, New Hampshire, patients have the option of group exercise classes, home exercise plans, and individual work with physical therapists at the hospital. In a recently released video about the program, Gary Schwartz, M.D., a medical oncologist at the Norris Cotton Cancer Center, emphasizes the value of cancer patients' exercise programs. The video profiles several breast cancer survivors and shows their use of simple exercise plans, which are supported by the physical therapists at the cancer center. Their exercise plans included aerobic and strength-training components.

Dr. Schwartz's list of mentioned benefits include: improving the speed of a patient's recovery from surgery; reducing recurrence rates; helping with osteoporosis; helping with lymphedema; reducing fatigue; helping with weight management, which helps with cancer prognosis; helping to control insulin levels optimally; and helping with range of motion affected by radiation therapy. Breast cancer patients in Dr. Schwartz's cancer treatment center are being supported by professionally managed physical therapy programs.

Another model for encouraging cancer patients to exercise finds hospitals and cancer centers partnering with fitness centers. An early leader was the Santa Barbara, California, program known as Well-Fit, which linked a cancer center's goals with the facilities of the Santa Barbara athletic club. The club offered programs free of charge, for a limited time, to cancer survivors.

Expanding on that model, the Center for Cancer Care at Exeter Hospital in Exeter, New Hampshire, helped to create a health and fitness facility on the hospital grounds. At the fitness center, physical therapists and trainers use the Well-Fit model to help cancer patients maintain strength and fitness during cancer treatment. They offer a twice-weekly program for twenty weeks to cancer patients. Individualized rehabilitation (physical therapy) sessions are also available. The staff has received training specific to oncology-related care.

Here is their own description of the program: "Cancer Well-Fit participants receive an individualized exercise program consisting of cardiovascular, strength training, and flexibility exercises, offering a comprehensive approach to fitness." The popularity of these cancer patient programs has led to increased numbers of cancer patients referred to and, ultimately, seeking care at the hospital. Hospitals and doctors have supported stress reduction and exercise programs for heart disease patients, smoking cessation for smokers, and weight reduction programs for diabetics. Acknowledging that everyday behaviors influence patient health is not new.

In the absence of extensive programs within their own facilities, some hospitals will partner with programs in the community that benefit patients. This could be as simple as referring a patient to a lymphedema expert for physical therapy. Or it could include informing patients of yoga, meditation, strength training, and other fitness programs available in the community. Sometimes these programs are run in separate non-profit facilities, such as at the YMCA, yoga centers, or private fitness centers. Other times, the offerings are linked to community home health and hospice organizations or cancer survivorship centers at non-profit organizations such as Gilda's Clubs.

Some hospitals or cancer centers partner with community programs that focus on survivorship care, which is the broad term used for issues that cancer survivors face after completion of cancer treatment. These hospitals acknowledge the benefits to patients and survivors of integrated wellness care and exercise.

One example is the Yale Cancer Center's affiliation with the Connecticut Challenge Survivorship Clinic. The Yale Cancer Center is a National Cancer Institute-designated cancer center, and the Connecticut Challenge Survivorship Clinic is a non-profit organization serving all of Connecticut.

On their website, they write: "The primary focus is on providing guidance and direction to empower survivors to take steps to maximize their health, quality of life, and longevity. Additionally, the team educates survivors on the prevention, detection, and treatment of complications resulting from cancer treatment." An oncologist, a nutritionist, an exercise therapist, and a social worker all work in collaboration in caring for patients. The program makes exercise and fitness recommendations for survivors.

TRAINING SPECIALISTS AND PLANNING FUTURE PROGRAMS

The physical therapists and others who are involved in cancer patient care at the Cancer Center at Exeter Hospital receive specialized training within their own facility. They also extend their two-day training to others from beyond their facility, reaching about seventy-five professionals each year. "The curriculum includes basic and advanced lectures from physicians, nurses, social workers, therapists and other oncology professionals in order to provide a solid foundation for our staff. Topics include medical oncology, radiation oncology, pathology, radiology, surgery, and end-of-life care. Special topics have included lymphedema, pain management, yoga, oncology massage, and spirituality." Their educational efforts also include site visits by visiting professionals and consulting.

The ACSM has recently established guidelines for certification for physical therapists in oncology care. In coordination with the American Cancer Society, they have established a core curriculum for certifying cancer exercise trainers (CETs) through education about issues in physical therapy for people in cancer recovery.

This new tier of certification will help establish a greater number of physical therapists who understand oncology-related issues as they overlap with exercise needs of people in cancer treatment and beyond. You can contact the American College of Sports Medicine to see if there are any certified CETs near you.

Additionally, an entrepreneurial consulting company has emerged, ready to help medical facilities design cancer center-based exercise programs and facilities. The company, Oncology Rehab Partners, states on their website in 2011 that they offer training for physical therapists and others, in oncology-rehab, as well as offering consultations to hospitals that are designing programs. They are trying to establish standards for oncology rehabilitation. This indicates that there is a significant commercial market for helping hospitals build professional programs in fitness for cancer patients. That reality bodes well for the future of exercise programs in cancer centers.

MODEL INTEGRATIVE CANCER CARE CENTERS

Let's look at leading innovative cancer centers that recognized the role of exercise in cancer treatment some years ago. The Block Center, a leading medical facility for integrative cancer care, run by Keith Block, M.D., in Evanston, Illinois, features exercise as a part of integrated cancer care. The Cancer Treatment Centers of America, which have several locations, also do the same. These institutions have not just added on integrative cancer care services. They began with the holistic approach that combines conventional medical treatment with caring for the whole patient and supporting their health in an integrated way.

Dr. Block's recent book, *Life Over Cancer*, details the holistic approach that defines integrative cancer care at the medical institution that he runs. Their website describes the program in this way: "The care provided a Block Center patient embodies the highest level of conventional medicine and integrates those conventional protocols with advanced complementary therapies that address the physical, nutritional, psychosocial, and spiritual aspects of healing and recovery."

The physical exercise program that is used at the Block Center uses a "strength-building, aerobic and Eastern training program." Each patient receives an individualized program based on his or her own specific condition. There are some elements of yoga, for "gentle stretches, strengthening poses and deep breathing techniques." Additionally, co-founders Dr. Block and his wife, Penny Block, developed a unique program that uses movement, stretching, and breathing elements, from both Eastern and Western traditions.

They call their program "Be-fit Bio-conditioning." It uses the same three elements of exercise that are traditionally considered to be necessary for strength and fitness: aerobic conditioning, strength training, and flexibility work. What is uniquely compelling is that Dr. Block, in his book, points out that it is his conviction that maintaining or improving the patient's physical fitness, at all points during cancer treatment—even among patients with poor prognoses or mobility limitations—is vital to patient outcome with cancer treatment.

Note: Dr. Block is lauded as "the guiding force in the world of integrative cancer treatment" by a respected authority from M.D. Anderson Cancer Center. I have no connection to him, but if I had a cancer recurrence, his cancer center would be on the top of my list. So, here is my advice: Go buy a copy of *Life Over Cancer*, which covers many topics in state-of-the-art integrated cancer care. If you add that book and *Anticancer* to your library, you will be well served regarding important topics other than exercise.

SHOULD YOU WAIT FOR MORE STUDIES?

Some of you would like to hear that your exact health status has been extensively studied. Breast cancer survivors are the group most studied for the effects of exercise on their status. However, unless you are a breast cancer survivor, the effects of exercise on your particular cancer may not have been studied extensively yet. It will take many years and much academic research before all the subcomponents can be picked apart. The studies will be slow to reach groups of patients who have less common cancers. Because exercise, as therapy, is so non-controversial, perhaps it is not important to wait for studies of your exact situation and diagnosis.

One aspect of exercise and cancer recovery is easy to overlook: the lack of argument against exercise. There is no significant disagreement about the idea that physical activity benefits cancer patients. After ASCM's expert panel analyzed 140 peer-reviewed clinical studies, no controversy about the benefits of exercise emerged. Few areas of medicine are this free of controversy. Yes, there are some precautions and considerations for individual cancer patients, which are discussed in the next three chapters, but there are no generalized problems with exercise during cancer recovery. Quite the opposite. In discussions about exercise during cancer recovery, there are only widely touted merits.

The expert panel on exercise and cancer found so little controversy about the merits of exercise for cancer patients that they underlined the axiom: <u>Avoid inactivity</u>. This advice is appropriate for people during cancer treatment and in other stages of cancer recovery, the panel said, with just a few considerations and some exceptions.

You should celebrate the lack of evidence against exercise. There is no indication of any generalized, pervasive risk to doing exercise for most cancer patients. This absence of conflict may seem like a small thing, but it is not.

TIPPING POINT

When I first conceived of writing this chapter, I planned to analyze the details of published, double-blind, clinical studies on exercise and cancer recovery, weighing nuanced claims with honest caution. I did not do that, as you have seen. After finding that a panel of qualified experts at the ACSM had already done it, I was delighted to present their conclusions instead.

Exercise programs for cancer patients are showing up at hospitals, cancer centers, and in community-supported programs. The presence of new certifications of cancer exercise trainers, the rise of businesses helping hospitals to integrate oncology-rehab care into their offerings, and other signs of acceptance for exercise-for-cancer-patients are too numerous to list here. Cancer centers with nationally prominent reputations either have, or likely soon will have, offerings in support of patients being active during cancer treatment. To find more information, make inquiries at your own treating facility.

It would appear that medicine has reached a tipping point where advising physical activity for cancer patients is mainstream and no longer questioned. Exercise benefits patients' overall health and their cancer recovery. Although no one can guarantee that your cancer will be cured, adding exercise to your cancer treatment helps your health and your cancer recovery. You can proceed to make your exercise plans in full confidence that medical professionals are behind you. In fact, it may be hard for future clinical studies to involve patients who are advised not to exercise because being inactive can hurt their recovery.

Don't wonder and don't wait. Be physically active against cancer!

CHAPTER THREE

YOUR DECISION TO BE ACTIVE AGAINST CANCER

Renowned oncologist Marisa Weiss, M.D., was recently interviewed on National Public Radio's program *Fresh Air* about her breast cancer experience. She is a noted breast cancer expert, a practicing physician, and the founder of the website called breast-cancer.org. A breast cancer survivor herself, Dr. Weiss remarked that she feels better now than she felt before she had cancer because she took her own medical advice. "I cleaned up my act," she said, by making the best self-care choices that she could.

Because Dr. Weiss faces a long-term risk of cancer recurrence, she "did everything that the doctors advised," but she also did more. She exercised; reduced her intake of pesticide-laden foods; lost body fat; reduced her stress; and committed herself to getting enough sleep. Her commitment to excellent, pro-active self-care choices, including exercise, was thrilling to hear. This relatively new sense of priorities will soon inform more medical practitioners involved in cancer care.

DO EVERYTHING: YOUR SELF-CARE CHOICES

Dr. Weiss appears to have the same perspective that I had during my cancer treatment: Do everything to heal and build health. First, of course, you should do everything that your doctors tell you to do in terms of your choices of surgery, chemotherapy, and radiation. Beyond that, though, do everything that is in the best interest of your long-term overall health. Self-care choices about nutrition, sleep, exercise and environmental exposures are not less important to your health simply because they are less overtly medical in nature and more under your complete daily control. If you want to optimally fight cancer, you need to use self-care strategies. Period. The jury is in: self-care matters.

Here is how I thought about this issue during my own cancer challenge. Even when I was able to show no evidence of disease (familiarly also known as NED) after surgery and chemotherapy, I also faced a long-term risk of recurrence. In fact, with my cancer type, I never will become cured. Accumulating time spent without evidence of disease and without recurrence will be my comfort, but I will never get a pass that says that my cancer cannot return.

For some of you, this is also the case. Others of you will be declared cured after a certain number of years. However, even for those of you who get a cure from your original cancer, you may face a risk of a different type of cancer. In fact, all of us, while alive, are at risk for cancer—and we are at relatively high risk, especially in the United States.

What I decided, when I was facing cancer treatment, is that I wanted to have no regrets. I wanted to "do everything." Perhaps this approach will resonate with some of you who are hedging about whether or not you need to go the extra mile. Approach any cancer crisis as if you want to have no regrets and do all that you can to improve your cancer recovery.

Has your cancer woken you up to the fact that there's no time to waste becoming as healthy as you can? Do you want to look back later and wonder if you should have done more for your health? Do everything that you can do. You can decide to throw the book at cancer and do everything that you can on behalf of your own health. Ask yourself, "Is there anything reasonable that I can do to lower my cancer risk?" Throw the book at cancer. Any book. This book!

COMMIT TO BEING ACTIVE

There's no time like the present to stay active. Now is the right time to commit to exercising for your own health, whether this time is early after your diagnosis, during your cancer treatment, or after your treatment has ended. While your cancer risk is anything but theoretical, it's a good time to be active. When you deeply appreciate how much good health means to you, it's a good time to exercise. When you are willing to change your lifestyle to save your health or your life, that's the right time to use exercise to beat cancer. While you are worried about your recovery or a recurrence, while you are trying to cope with chemotherapy, or while you are trying to get back a sense of normal living: Exercise for the sake of your health.

Try this statement: "I commit to exercising a small amount, daily, during my cancer treatment as a way to help recover my health. I do this out of love for my life and a desire to be healthy again. I will embrace exercise in the amounts and types that I can do. I will start today."

Don't you feel better already? Make the commitment to begin to exercise and then begin. Begin today with a short walk, if you are comfortable with that. You are being active in order to fight against cancer. Those of us who have already signed up for things such as arduous chemotherapy or radiation have to be encouraged. In comparison to those treatment choices, signing up for exercise is a wonderful thing.

When you prescribe regular exercise for yourself, you will be aligning yourself with leading medical doctors, current medical research, and many cancer treatment programs at leading cancer hospitals, as well as with programs by Livestrong and other cancer advocacy organizations. Make the commitment to be active against cancer today.

EXERCISE STRATEGY: ONE DAY AT A TIME

After you have made your commitment to exercise, then take it one day a time as you begin. Some of you may want to make no decision to exercise. You may want to procrastinate. You may want to hedge, but postponing the decision to exercise is actually the same as not exercising. Please don't be passive and let the chance to be physically active pass you by.

Honestly, there are really only two choices: decide to exercise the best you can or decide not to exercise. It's not hard to tell which group you are in. If you are in the non-exercising group, and you want to change, keep reading. If you repeatedly resolve to be more active, but you fail to do so, you might need more support emotionally for it. You could talk with a counselor about your resistance to exercise. Ask for whatever help you might need. I hope reading this book will work for you!

For now, though, I'll assume that you just need the information on what to do and how to do it. Make the decision that will reward your health: exercise. Let's get started finding an exercise plan that fits you today!

Use exercise to remind yourself that you are in charge of protecting your own health as much as you can. When I am able to exercise daily, I know that I am taking care of myself and helping my health status. You can use exercise to support good health. By being in touch with your fitness and strength each day, you can help to keep up with self-care habits. Being active also tends to make it easier to regulate your eating and sleeping habits, two other big contributors to your health.

EXERCISE IS NATURAL FOR HUMANS

Keep your reasons to exercise simple. We are animals and not meant to be sedentary ones. Activity is natural and helpful to our bodies. Apparently, this is true even if you have had or have cancer. Trust the common sense advice to stay as active as appropriate while you are in a cancer challenge.

If you are a seasoned athlete, you already know the physical sense of satisfaction that comes from being active. If that satisfaction is new to you, please know that you can build up to achieving it. Have you ever watched The Biggest Loser, which documents people's successful efforts to lose a lot of weight? I love to see the transformation of people's spirits—and health—as they become more fit and more accustomed to exercise. I believe that exercise can help turn around anyone's health and life. Exercise is just natural in a way that sitting at a desk, in a car, or on our couches all day is not. You know it and I know it. This is a good time to act like your life depends on it!

YOU CAN BE YOUR OWN EXPERT

Exercise is not so technical that you can't add a meaningful dose of exercise to your life on your own. With some instruction, if needed, and approval from your doctor, you can exercise. You can do it for free, if you want to choose certain activities. You can exercise at home. You can modify activity levels to suit your ups and downs. Best of all, you can reap all the benefits of exercise without a nurse, surgeon, or extra hospital visit.

"BUT I HATE TO EXERCISE..."

If exercise is not something that you like, please just keep reading. This book has been written with you in mind, and its many tips can help you enjoy or, at least, tolerate exercise. You may also be inspired by the profiles of cancer survivors. When I read through the profiles, I admire their courage and commitment.

I hate cancer. I hate losing friends and family to cancer. I hate seeing that children die of cancer. I hate the increasing rates of cancer. Maybe it's okay to hate these things or, perhaps, dislike them. But hating to exercise? Do you really have time for that?

BEFORE AND AFTER YOUR CANCER DIAGNOSIS

For some of you, regular exercise will be a change from your pre-cancer lifestyle. If that's the case, you might be flexible about which type of exercise to do during your cancer recovery. You can learn the joys and benefits of exercise as you use activities to help you heal from cancer, while gaining strength and fitness.

If you were an athletic person or an athlete before cancer, you have the benefit of your past experience of sports and activities. However, as an athletic person, you may experience a sense of loss or frustration if you cannot continue your usual athletic activities during cancer treatment. You may be able to do some of your favorite sports, but you might need to do them at a much reduced pace or intensity. Or you may have to switch activities. You may need some time to adjust to your body's limitations or changes during or after cancer treatment.

Perhaps you can think of any of your new cancer-related limitations as very bizarre sports injuries. Like with sports injuries, you need to adjust your activities to suit your condition while you heal. Of course, cancer is different than injuries, but the process is the same: trying to adapt to limitations, work around them, and still get exercise.

GOOD HEALTH IS YOUR TOP GOAL

If you are in recovery from cancer, you no doubt want to get your good health status back. Your motivation for exercise can be very clear: you want to exercise in order to regain your health. Regaining your good health trumps any other exercise goal, so your exercise plans will reflect this basic goal. You're not exercising during cancer recovery primarily to have fun or even to maintain a certain fitness level or performance in sports.

Having your health as your highest priority may mean letting go of other goals if you are in the habit of enjoying a lot of physical activities and sports. Although it may be disappointing at first, cancer requires a lot of adjustments. The good news is that you can probably continue to exercise a significant amount. You can be very motivated by an exercise plan that directly supports your goal of conquering cancer.

Ultimately, regaining your health after cancer can feel like the most meaningful exercise goal that you have ever had. And, after the wonderful day when the doctor says, "See you in three months," exercise can still be there for you every day.

CHAPTER FOUR

TALK WITH YOUR DOCTOR ABOUT YOUR ACTIVITIES

P lease check with your treating doctor or medical team about your plans to exercise during your cancer recovery. Although this book provides a lot of information, only you and your medical team know your own health situation in depth. Start your exercise program only after you get medical advice from your own medical doctor. This book cannot offer personalized medical advice for you and your exact condition. You will want to ask your medical caregivers about any particular restrictions, concerns, or advice that they might have. Ask them what type of exercise they recommend for you, what activities they might recommend against, and what your special medical issues, if any, might be. Ideally, they will have answers to your exercise-related and treatment-related questions.

Remember, during your cancer treatment and recovery, your condition is best known to your treating medical professionals. No one knows your health history as well as you and your medical team. There are hundreds of chemotherapeutic agents, many varied radiologic regimens, surgeries, disease subtypes, and pre-existing conditions in cancer treatment. Use this book only as a starting point for your decisions and as guidance. Get all the information that you need for your particular health status, and be aware that your health status may change over time. Continue with your exercise plans only as long as your medical team agrees with your exercise choices.

Sometimes you will easily get all the information you need from your medical team, but other times you may be left with questions. Perhaps exercise is outside of what your doctor feels comfortable discussing as a professional. Doctors, generally, are not fond of speculation or of giving non-expert advice. If your doctor is not able to advise you well about exercise and you need more guidance, feel free to ask your doctor to recommend someone else who can help you. If you still have unanswered questions, you might ask for a referral to a physical therapist or a sports medicine professional for information. Ask if there are any professionals in your community who work well with people in cancer recovery.

SEEK MORE ADVICE, IF NEEDED

Another way to find information is through reaching out to the community of survivors of your type of cancer. You can find communities online or in the real world, at cancer-fundraising events, or through networking. You can make contact with the American Cancer Society, Livestrong, Gilda's clubs, your local medical center's cancer outreach programs, or other local or national organizations. See the resources section at the end of this book for some ideas.

You should be careful not to mistake anecdotes for medical guidance, but sometimes you can get help from fellow survivors. They may simply help direct you to local medical professionals who can answer your questions.

How do you know whom to trust? It's not always easy. Some-times your doctor is terrific at surgery and chemotherapy but not very knowledgeable about exercise's impact on your condition. Some doctors may make general and vague statements, which may discourage you. Formerly, many physicians were apt to give only this general advice to cancer patients: "Take it easy. Don't push yourself to exercise." If you think your doctor is just generally negative about exercise, respectfully ask if he or she can be more specific about their exact concerns. You can always ask for your doctor's reasoning if you feel that the explanations are too vague, ambiguous or too general.

If your doctor is neutral or indifferent about your exercise plans, ask about finding other resources for you in the medical center or community. There may be someone else on the medical staff that might have more information for you regarding your exercise options. If you are respectful in your requests for help, you should receive good answers.

BE SPECIFIC IN YOUR DISCUSSIONS

Perhaps you need to tell your doctor your specific exercise plans. If you have practical or medical concerns, such as unfamiliarity with using weights or a concern about your heart's condition, ask questions. On their side, the physician may have some very specific medical concerns for you, such as bone metastases that weaken your bones' strength. Ideally, you should be able to discuss your concerns and your doctor should be able to discuss his or her own.

If a physician is negative about your prospects for exercise, suggest that you both discuss your plans as specifically as possible. Don't just suggest that you want to do "a lot of exercise" during treatment. Spell it out. For example, say that you want to walk for 15 minutes for 5 days per week and build up your strength again. Sometimes your doctor may be worried that you are going to try to run a marathon without training, while anemic, or when you are ill prepared. Keep your communication brief, but open and thorough.

If you don't yet have exact plans to discuss, ask about the following possibility. Ask if there are any restrictions for you regarding starting a program of daily walking for 10 to 30 minutes at a comfortable pace. Explain that you may ask more questions later. Further chapters in this book will help you choose from a range of good activity choices, and you can run these choices by your doctor as you begin.

Keep a respectful tone, understand the limitations of your short medical appointments, and then, take a pro-active approach to getting the information that you need. You can do it! Exercise, luckily, is not overly technical. You should be able to get the answers to your questions from the right medical authorities, and feel confident in your exercise plans.

USE YOUR BODY'S INTUITION

Eventually, you can learn to trust yourself, your body's feedback, and how you feel when you do light to moderate exercise. When you are going through cancer treatment, don't try to be some kind of super-athlete or hero. Never try to withstand significant pain or ignore things that would make a normal person stop exercising such as dizziness, fever, or intense nausea. (There are more detailed warnings about contraindications to exercise in the next chapter.)

When you try to judge the effects, immediately, of exercise, at the very least, please use the "reasonable person test." What would a reasonable person do? Go for a long run when dehydrated after a night of no rest and upset stomach? No. That's not a reasonable choice. Do not be so attached to the idea of a certain exercise plan that you refuse to listen to your body's signals to stop. Chapter ten will show you many choices for modifying your exercise plans according to your day-to-day condition.

What can be difficult, especially with some chemotherapies and radiation, is sorting out the minor complaints that are safe to ignore from the physical symptoms that you should not ignore.

Cancer treatments produce many unusual side effects that you'll need to sort out as they come up. Ask your chemo nurse, an experienced physical therapist, or other expert to help you sort out your specific issues. Further medical guidance is in chapters five and ten of this book; use that to help yourself have an educated discussion with your caregivers.

Comparing your experience to that of other patients is sometimes helpful and sometimes misleading. I think of my own example. Because I was a lifelong endurance athlete before my illness and treatment, I was able to do a six-hour hike despite some of my chemotherapy's side effects. I had a good baseline of fitness, an ability to judge my fatigue, and good leg strength. However, my activity choice would not be appropriate for many other patients. If you had been leading a fairly inactive lifestyle at the time of your illness, you might want to start a gentle walking program that expands slowly over time. Do what is appropriate for you.

Compare notes with people if you like, but always keep in mind that your situation may be different as far as base conditioning, cancer progression, drug side effects, and blood counts. More is not better; appropriate is better when it comes to exercise during cancer treatment—and probably any other time!

REMEMBER WHY YOU CHOSE YOUR DOCTORS

As a last note, I want to suggest that even if your exercise plans are very important to you during your cancer treatment, you don't need to choose your surgeon, medical oncologist, or radiation oncologist by their exercise expertise. Remember, you have chosen your doctor and team for their credentials in cancer care. I wouldn't change doctors because they weren't on board with my exercise plans if I liked them for their cancer-treating skills. Gaining support about exercise from your treating physicians might be helpful, but it's not always the most crucial aspect of their medical care of you.

Exercise, like walking or stretching, is not difficult in concept or in the doing. You don't always need a medical advisor to fine-tune your exercise programs. Keep faith in your doctors for their specialized knowledge and skills in cancer care. You can keep them informed about your exercise activities, if you have any medical questions as you go on.

CHAPTER FIVE

WHEN NOT TO EXERCISE: CONTRAINDICATIONS

"Contraindicated" is a word that is familiar to all doctors, but it may not be familiar to you. If an activity is contraindicated, it means that you should not do that activity because it would have negative consequences for your health. When a certain drug is contraindicated for high blood pressure, for example, it means that you should not take it if you have high blood pressure. The contraindicated medication might make your high blood pressure worse, and that's not good!

If an intense weight-lifting program is contraindicated when you have bone metastases, it means that you should not do heavy weight lifting. In that example, the danger is a significant risk of bone fractures because your bones are not completely healthy and strong.

Physicians are well trained to think in terms of contraindications. Contraindications are like stop signs on the road to health. Identifying contraindications is very important. When you ask about doing a certain exercise activity, doctors may think first:

"What harm would it do to the patient's health?" If, in their minds, the risks are too great, then they will see the activity as contraindicated.

In the absence of contraindications, you will likely get the go-ahead from your physician to do moderate exercise. Even without studies that have measured the impact of exercise regimens similar to the one you are proposing, if the doctor sees no contraindications, you may get the green light.

Let's look at some common contraindications for exercise during cancer treatment. Using American Cancer Society guidelines and the *Exercise Guidelines for Cancer Survivors* by ACSM as our sources, here are some of the known important contraindications for exercise for cancer patients. Some of the contraindications are particular to cancer patients, although others apply to all people.

SYMPTOMS OR SIGNS TO STOP EXERCISING

1. If you are in severe pain, have a fever, or are very weak, do not attempt to exercise.

2. Do not exercise if you are dehydrated from recent vomiting, diarrhea, or another cause. Wait until 24 to 48 hours after you are able to hold food in normally before exercising to assure that your electrolyte balance is restored to normal. If you are in doubt about whether or not you are dehydrated, do not exercise. Discuss your condition with your medical team first.

3. Stop exercising if at any time you feel faint or dizzy. You may lose your balance, fall, and get injured. Play it safe.

4. Stop exercising if you have a very high or unusual heart rate, an irregular heartbeat, palpitations, pain in your chest, pain down your arm, sudden nausea, sweating, or dizziness that may be related to a heart episode. If you think you are having a heart attack, call 911 and get medical attention.

5. Stop exercising if you feel nauseated from pain or light-headed from the effort to exercise.

6. If you develop redness, swelling, or sudden pain in your lower leg, stop exercising and seek medical attention. You may have a blood clot that can travel to your heart and lungs, causing sudden death (pulmonary embolism).

7. You can expect to be instructed by your doctor to avoid any strenuous exercise for six weeks after a surgical event. If the doctor's meaning is not clear enough to you, ask for more details. For example, early exercise following an abdominal surgery can lead to an incisional hernia, no matter how good your pre-surgery conditioning was. Don't confuse your fitness level with your readiness for activity in the first six weeks after surgery. Do not assume during the first six weeks that you can do any strength workouts, weight lifting, running or other sustained aerobic efforts, or swimming.

In general, do not assume anything in the first six weeks post-surgery. If you have questions, call your doctor's office. The only foolish questions right after surgery are the ones that you don't ask. Follow your doctor's advice to the "T." Before resuming your exercise activities, get clearance at your six-week follow-up visit with your doctor.

OTHER CONCERNS FOR SOME CANCER SURVIVORS

1. If you are receiving or have received radiation treatments, your affected bones may have an increased risk of fractures if you lift heavy weight or do intense weight-bearing high-impact activity, depending on where the radiation was. On the other hand, bone integ-

rity is aided by improved muscle strength and tone, so appropriate exercise can help prevent fractures. Ask your doctor for specific advise before choosing your activities so that they are appropriate to you.

2. If you have metastatic cancer, ask your doctor before beginning any exercise program. Certain exercise choices may not be appropriate, depending on the location of the metastases. For example, if you have bone metastases, you likely have increased risk of fractures, as described above. Also, if you have metastatic cancer, you may have bone metastases that are not yet documented or known. Ask your doctor about any concerns. Choosing flexibility activities, low-impact activities or resistance-band use may be appropriate. Get guidance for yourself from a physical therapist experienced with cancer patients or other knowledgeable professionals.

3. If you have a brain tumor or tumors, do not do vigorous aerobic exercise without physician approval, as such exercise is likely to be contraindicated. You may be at risk of seizures that could cause you to slip and fall, or have worse effects.

4. Ask your physician what your restrictions might be if you have an infusion port in your chest. Contact sports are contraindicated.

5. Minimize infection if you have a catheter in place, by avoiding water or other exposures to infection. Ask your doctor for guidance.

ADDITIONAL PRECAUTIONS

The following precautions from the ACSM affect fewer people, but if you have any of these concerns, discuss them with your treating medical team.

1. If you have had an ostomy, make sure infection prevention controls are adequate.

2. If you are at risk of a hernia, do not undertake weight lifting without supervision and avoid heavy weights.

3. If you have lower-body lymphedema from gyneco-logical surgery, seek medical advice about swelling and exercise. You may be able to use compression wear beneficially or you may have some limitations on your activities.

4. If you have been treated with ADT, consider yourself at risk for bone fractures and seek medical advice.

5. If you have had an ostomy, do not attempt contact sports without getting medical advice. They may be contraindicated.

6. If you have received radiation, your skin may be irritated by the kinds of chemicals used in pools or hot tubs. Stay out of pools and hot tubs, unless your radiation oncologist helps you to make appropriate accommodations.

7. If you are obese, have arthritis, or have pre-existing physical disabilities, work with a trained medical professional, physical therapists or other professionals for guidance about exercise.

ASK FOR HELP

Remember, knowledge is power, so the more that you know about your condition, the better your choices can be. You should be able to get careful, complete explanations from your doctor, your nurses, and other professionals, as well as by doing your own research. Many organizations exist in support of survivors of particular cancers, and they may provide access to counselors or others who can help you build up your knowledge of your cancer's issues.

All throughout the experience of cancer recovery remember that you always have the right to try to understand the medical implications of your treatment by your medical team. If you feel overwhelmed or confused, ask for more help. Most cancer professionals know how to help you find the right resources. Cancer is difficult enough, as an experience. Ask for the support that you need so that you can understand as much as you want to about it.

CHAPTER SIX

BE ACTIVE AGAINST CANCER: CHOOSE A PLAN

A cancer challenge is a personal crisis. When you received your cancer diagnosis, you had many crucial concerns all at once. Although no two people go through a cancer challenge exactly the same, most people find that it shakes up their sense of priorities. What is important in your life can become very obvious. What is missing from your life can also be obvious. Has taking care of your body with adequate exercise been part of your life? Whether you had the best exercise habits before your cancer diagnosis or had habitually avoided being active, now is the time to reconsider exercise. Let's formulate a plan for you.

If you look forward to exercise as being fun and a relief from cancer troubles, that's great. If you dread exercise, but you're willing to do it—well, that's good enough. Do whatever it takes to start being active. You can learn to love your exercise adventures, but, for now, just make a commitment to begin exercising.

Here is a note for those of you who are turned off at the very mention of an exercise plan. Maybe you don't want to schedule your physical activities. Maybe you think that if you make an exercise plan, exercise will take over your life or the plan will be too restricting. Please be encouraged. You can make very simple, flexible, satisfying, and personalized plans. There will be many tips to help you succeed, and you can adjust the plans to fit your needs. I have included a whole chapter on making such adjustments.

Besides, if you have no exercise plan at all... well, what's your plan? You're not likely to do routine, regular exercise without a plan. Put your physical activities on your schedule of your days or don't expect to be consistent with them. Bear with me: Exercise planning can be empowering, especially when you're using exercise to help your cancer recovery.

In this chapter, I am introducing the two types of plans and giving some background information about exercise types. The full exercise plans are in the next two chapters.

STARTING PLAN: NURTURE THE HABIT OF BEING ACTIVE

The Starting Plan is for those who have not exercised regularly in the last three to six weeks or longer. Perhaps you needed to stop exercising due to side effects or surgery. Perhaps you are currently out of the habit of regular exercise. Begin with the Starting Plan if you have had a significant lay-off from exercise, even if you are fairly fit. You can progress out of the Starting Plan smoothly into the next plan, the Sustaining Plan.

Remember, there's no shame in starting here. If your health has been disrupted, it's better to ease back into exercise gradually and consistently than to try to go back immediately to what you were doing before the disruption. You don't need a sports injury to compound your health challenges.

Within this group, many levels of fitness are represented, but you will tailor the Starting Plan to your condition at the outset. It's fine to be in this group if you have some restrictions to your exercise. You may be starting new cancer treatment, receiving cancer treatment, ending treatment, or have had cancer in the past.

With the Starting Plan, you will develop a habit of exercise. It's the foundation upon which you will build. The emphasis is on building the habit of exercise, not doing the most activity that you can. Many people fail to exercise because they push too hard at first and get discouraged. The Starting Plan helps you avoid that pitfall.

SUSTAINING PLAN: OPTIMAL ACTIVITIES

The Sustaining Plan will help you to do aerobic exercise for a minimum of 30 to 45 minutes, five days per week, plus strength and flexibility workouts. You can benefit from sustaining these levels of exercise indefinitely. The Sustaining Plan also helps you fine-tune your exercise plans so that they will serve you well in the long term. The Sustaining Plan presents ways to personalize your plan, keep motivated, and add various activities to keep exercise interesting… and fun.

ADJUSTING YOUR ACTIVITY PLANS

An entire chapter will present adjustments to your exercise plans to use when you can't always do your ideal schedule. The many contingency strategies will be useful to many people in active cancer treatment. The slogan of the adjustments to plans could be: "Some exercise is better than no exercise." Cancer surgery, cancer treatment, or other aspects of cancer may reduce your ability to exercise at your best level. However, you can exercise with modified goals that include boosting your immune system function, tolerating treatment better, and improving your sleep, digestion, or energy levels. Even small, frequent amounts of exercise can make a great difference to you, both physically and emotionally. Plus, if you make appropriate adjustments, you can keep thinking of yourself as having an exercise plan, even if there are days when you cannot exercise very much or at all.

You may progress from one plan to another over time. For example, you may already have been exercising when you suddenly needed a cancer surgery. You were unable to exercise very much for several weeks as a result, so you might find yourself using the Starting Plan as you begin to exercise again. You may then recover some of your fitness and stamina so that you can move to the Sustaining Plan. Later, as you undergo chemotherapy, you may need to make adjustments to your plan as your energy level drops.

THE THREE TYPES OF EXERCISE

Most types of activity fall in to one of these categories of exercise: aerobic activity, strength training, and flexibility. If you want to best support your health with exercise, first understand these three components. You'll incorporate each of these types of activities into whatever plan you make.

Aerobic Fitness

Aerobic fitness is what many people think of as exercise, but it is actually the type of exercise that makes your heart pump blood more vigorously through your body. Your increased breathing rate makes your lungs bring more oxygen into your circulating blood. As a result, blood delivers the amount of oxygen that your muscles need to do their work.

Aerobic exercise is also sometimes called cardiopulmonary exercise, which emphasizes the heart and lung activities. "Cardio" means heart-related and "pulmonary" means lung-related. Sometimes, aerobic exercise is just called "cardio" or "cardiovascular," where vascular refers to your blood vessels.

Most of us know what it feels like to do aerobic exercise if we simply walk fast enough to speed up our heart rate and our breathing. You don't have to be racing to do aerobic exercise.

Aerobics classes, which are fitness classes involving dance steps and music, are popular. They are easy enough for many non-athletes and difficult enough to lead to improvements in fitness levels.

Perhaps you have had the experience of running as fast as you can until you come up short of breath with a heavy, tired feeling in your legs. This is anaerobic exercise: your heart-lung system cannot deliver oxygen fast enough for the demands that you are putting on your muscles, so your muscles lack the oxygen they need to keep contracting to do work. Anaerobic exercise can be purposeful when you are trying to gain certain kinds of fitness, but it is beyond the scope of this book. Aerobic fitness is what we are after for your health.

Improving your aerobic conditioning takes time, but you are well rewarded with fitness gains. The body is very responsive to improvements in aerobic capacity. How do you improve your aerobic fitness? Practice, practice, practice.

If you watch a running race, the runners clearly illustrate differences in aerobic conditioning. One person's race pace might be easy for them when they run one mile in 6 minutes while another person can only run one mile in 12 minutes. Another person may not even be able to run a mile in 12 minutes, but he or she can walk quickly and cover a mile in 15 minutes at an aerobic pace.

In race results, mindset, strength, body composition, technique, and genetics are involved in different performances, but it is aerobic fitness that accounts for most of the observable differences in pace. Most recreational running racers know that doing more aerobic training equals racing faster.

The more aerobic fitness that you have, the easier it is for your blood to circulate efficiently and fire your muscles with oxygen. It also becomes easier for you to not tire with sustained exercise. Athletes who are distance runners, long-distance triathletes, cross-country ski racers, and cyclists are some of the best specimens of aerobically fit athletes. You don't have to have world-class goals to make gains in your aerobic fitness. All you need to do is work at it.

Some really good news: You can make dramatic gains in aerobic fitness in three to six weeks! Aerobic training doesn't have to be painful and exercise doesn't have to take over your life. If you have never worked on becoming more fit, consistently, you will be heartened to know that making gains in your aerobic fitness levels is as simple as doing more exercise with a raised pulse. It's a lot of fun to be aerobically fit.

Strength Training

Stronger muscles do more work more easily. To get stronger, you do things that use your muscles. If you want to generally tone muscles, you don't need to challenge them with heavy weights. If you do some weight-lifting activity with lighter weights, you can achieve meaningful results. You can even use your body as the weight, such as when doing yoga poses like "downward-facing dog," where you support your body weight on your arms.

Our muscles will get stronger based on what activities we do. Muscles, wonderfully, respond to challenges we present them by trying to get stronger. They just need the right challenges at the right times, and they will respond. It's easy to figure out what you can do to get stronger.

There is more good news here. It's never too late to start to get stronger. If you have not worked to become stronger in many years, your muscles will still respond to new challenges and gain strength. Strengthening your muscles usually goes together with building better bones, and it often goes together with losing body fat. Your resting metabolism, which is how your body operates itself at rest, is raised if you have more muscle mass. The translation: You can burn more calories at rest if you have stronger and bigger muscles. This is an attractive feature of being strong!

Flexibility

Flexibility is like the poor relative of the first two elements. It's the last to be thought of—unless you're a ballet dancer, a gymnast, a yogi, or you once had a good athletic coach. Flexibility is based on the ability of your muscles to relax or "return to length." Muscles do only two things: they contract (shorten) when you use the muscle to do work or they return to their un-contracted length. There are definite advantages to lengthening your muscles even if you don't want to be able to do ballet moves.

In order to do work, a muscle needs to contract. If the muscle is already in a state of being shortened or tight, you have lost some of that muscle's power. The more length that a muscle has habitually, the more easily you can use its full strength and power. This is what many athletes accomplish by warming up and then stretching: they are maximizing the work their muscles can do.

Other problems with inflexibility include pulling joints out of position or your spine out of alignment. Inflexibility can cause undue tension or discomfort. A good session of stretching can bring blood to the muscles in a way that feels good. Better flexibility can lead to general sense of well being, improved posture, and better movement patterns. Yoga combines strengthening with flexibility work for a potent mix of benefits.

The current thinking is that you should not do aggressive stretching before warming up your muscles. Always try to do 5 minutes of some activity like walking before stretching. The reason: trying to stretch a muscle that has been inactive may lead to undue stress on tendons. Trying to stretch muscles that are cold is less effective.

In each of the exercise plans in this book, there are recommendations for aerobic conditioning, strength training, and flexibility work. It's important to address each of the three in your overall exercise plans. Keeping all three in mind will help prevent injury, help you feel fit, gain muscle, feel relaxed, and reap many benefits of exercise.

With this basic understanding of aerobic fitness, strength work, and flexibility, let's get started on the specific plans for your exercise routine.

PROFILES OF INSPIRING SURVIVORS

Each of the remaining chapters concludes with a profile of a cancer survivor who used exercise in their healing. Some of these survivors did ordinary exercise, such as walking or going to the gym, but all of the survivors are also quietly extraordinary. These cancer survivors did their workouts with conviction, dedication, and commitment. Most of them kept up with exercise during cancer treatment with modifications of their previous activities. Their attitudes toward taking care of themselves with exercise made their entire cancer ordeals easier.

If you lack inspiration at any point, skip ahead to read these profiles. Some of the stories will astonish you, but even the more modest stories have the power to help you get moving. I believe all of them can give you hope. Enjoy.

※ ※ ※

ACTIVE SURVIVOR PROFILE: KRISTEN

SIGNING UP TO STAY HEALTHY

Kristen Harris, a wife and mother, was surprised by her breast cancer diagnosis at forty years old. She was in shape, active outdoors, and working full-time in Colorado. When she thinks back on her time with breast cancer, she summarizes like this: "You can't take your health for granted. You have to take care of your body." Kristen took an active stand for her health's sake before, during, and after her cancer treatment. Two years after her diagnosis, she recounted her story for me.

Kristen's cancer was diagnosed early and she had an excellent prognosis. Her friends were immediately asking her what they could do to help. "I want you all to come to the Romp to Stomp with me, "she told them.

Kristen had learned about the snowshoe and fundraising event, which raises money to fight breast cancer, by looking online. She had signed up immediately. Having both skied and snowshoed with her family for years, the outdoor winter event appealed to her. And, ideally, she thought, it was scheduled nearby in Frisco, Colorado, for ten days after her surgery. Her friends also signed up when she asked them and they helped her raise money.

The Romp to Stomp, where Kristen snowshoed five kilometers with her group, was so meaningful to her that she says now, "I'll do that event every year for as long as I can." It brought her friends and family around her, and one of her friends has become a superstar of fundraising for the event.

Following Kristen's surgical recovery, she gathered several opinions from medical doctors and decided to take their advice to receive five weeks of radiation. She continued working and she set a new exercise goal. She signed up for the Tri for the Cure, a triathlon event of five kilometers of running, one-half mile of swimming, and twelve miles of bike riding. Her plan was pretty simple: work, get radiation during the day, and train in the late afternoon. She tried to do one activity of the three–biking, running, or swimming–every day.

Having been told that radiation would make her feel yucky and tired, Kristen was happy to be having a different type of experience. She felt pretty good. She felt that the exercise helped her immensely, both mentally and physically. Her radiation oncologist was encouraged: "Keep doing what you're doing." He was the only medical doctor that she interacted with who promoted exercise to her. She healed quickly, within a few weeks after radiation ended.

At the Tri for the Cure, the cancer survivors wore pink caps. She met a lot of other survivors, including one who had been diagnosed at the same time as Kristen. The two women became friends. Her race went well: She completed the course in just over two hours.

Kristen started doing more yoga after an ankle injury. She found a group yoga class for cancer survivors, where the group offered some emotional support as well as yoga practice. Although she hasn't continued that class because of the distance from her home, she feels it was worthwhile. Yoga has helped in the shift she made with her exercise focus.

Currently, Kristen's usual method is to allot an hour for exercise, with five minutes to get her workout's outfit and her shoes on. Then for 45 minutes, she sweats. She walks or uses a stationary bike, lift weights, or does other activity. She allows some time at the end for a 10-minute cool-down and some stretching and relaxing.

As Kristen describes it, "Before cancer, I focused on wellness and feeling good. If I moved, I knew that I would feel better. Then, working out became about balance and walking away from the stresses of life to take time for me. Now, it's about peace and balance, not necessarily pushing myself, but protecting myself and keeping my body in balance. Exercise is not a burden. It's a way of being." Kristen continues to support Romp to Stomp and be grateful for her health.

CHAPTER SEVEN

THE STARTING PLAN: THE HABIT OF BEING ACTIVE

With the Starting Plan, you will adopt the good habit of exercising nearly every day. Your main challenge is showing up. Exactly what you do for exercise initially is not as important as getting accustomed to doing some exercise most days.

I think of fitness like this: You either exercise routinely or you don't. The goal of the Starting Plan is to get you into the group that does routine, frequent exercise. Simple as that. You can make it seem more complicated, but if you fail to do routine regular exercise, then you are not getting enough exercise. In contrast, there's a wonderful feeling that I have at the end of a day, knowing that I did my best to be active that day. Here's an easy program to help you get the exercise habit and stay with it.

STARTING PLAN SUMMARY

1. Do an aerobic activity, such as walking for 10 or 20 minutes per day, 6 days per week. Choose your initial number of minutes based on what is comfortable for you.

2. Progress to 30 minutes of aerobic exercise. Do this by exercising for three weeks at your starting level, then adding 5 minutes per day for 2 weeks. Then add another 5 minutes, if needed, in the same pattern, until you reach 30 minutes per day.

3. Do 30 minutes to 60 minutes of yoga once per week. Do easy poses and do not strain. You can mix in gentle stretching, as well.

4. Do the simple-at-home strength plan once per week or substitute your own strengthening program using the suggestions here.

WALKING AS YOUR AEROBIC ACTIVITY

Use walking as your basic aerobic activity, if you are starting to exercise and you are able to walk. Walking is free, simple, fulfilling, and easy. You can walk outdoors or indoors with a treadmill or in a mall. You can walk alone, with others, or with your dog. You can easily vary the speed, distance, and intensity.

Walking is a natural everyday movement. You already know how. It's easy to vary the pace. Walking builds fitness and it can lead easily into running or bike riding. You're not likely to get hurt if you are beginning a walking program without much fitness base.

Until you reach your goal of 30-minute periods of aerobic exercise, stay with walking as your main activity if you can. Why? You are building a habit and it is best to keep the mode of exercise the same for now. Also, you are not likely to get hurt doing your walks; you are building cardiovascular fitness. Walking is an easy habit to enjoy for most people.

ALTERNATIVES TO WALKING

If walking doesn't make sense as your choice, identify another aerobic sport. You could try swimming, swim aerobics classes, or bike riding (stationary or outdoor). You could dance: tap, jazz, ballet or modern; folk, hip-hop, or square. While watching a DVD, you can do workouts led by instructors in many different activities. Alternatively, you can hike on trails or go to a gym to use elliptical trainers, rowing machines, or other equipment.

When choosing, try to pick something that really appeals to you, is convenient, and affordable. It's important to set yourself up for success on all three of those levels. Put some time into deciding what will work for your lifestyle and interests.

If affordability is a big issue, get creative. You may want to invest some money for home equipment rather than getting a fitness club membership. A stationary bike can often be found on Craigslist for not much money, and if you have a bike in your house, it will always be available. Alternatively, find out if your local club or YMCA has any special membership rates for cancer survivors. Some offer special rates for cancer survivors for a period of time. Perhaps your hospital may be able to send you to a gym through physical therapy.

Choose an activity that you will enjoy. Some of you would prefer to go to a gym and do your workouts around other people. You might feel more secure and safer, and that's fine. Or you may enjoy using an exercise machine so that you can be seated, if, for example, you have balance problems. Or you might like having your workouts indoors at home so that you don't have to travel anywhere. Some people have better luck than others sticking with exercise at home. Sometimes the key is setting a regular time for it.

Note: Please don't start with running as your main activity if you are not already a runner or if the intensity would be too great for your current condition. Start with walking instead. It is too easy to get discouraged or injured with running if you try to do too much too soon. Transitioning from a walking program to running will be safer and more successful after a month or more of walking.

Also, if you are having many issues with side effects of treatment, stay with walking until your recovery is more advanced. For details on changing from a walking program to a running program, see the next chapter.

HOW OFTEN?

The ACSM's *Exercise Guidelines for Cancer Survivors* suggest that you get thirty minutes of aerobic exercise, five days a week. I would suggest that you exercise six days per week, but you are welcome to stick with five days if you really want to. Let me explain my thinking.

I strongly believe that if you want to exercise, you had best make it a daily habit. It will be easier to exercise consistently if you do it every day. You can take one day off from aerobic activities for a change. However, if you limit yourself to exercising just five days per week, then you have two days without your regular aerobic efforts. If you skip your aerobic activity just one extra time per week, you will be down to only four days in a week. That's a slippery slope. Your program can start to fall apart quickly. Before you know it, you have to work hard in order to get back in the groove.

Instead, plan to take only one day off from your aerobic routine and do your flexibility work that day. You'll be maintaining the habit of exercising every day. If you can make exercise a habit, it will be so much easier to accomplish. If you exercise every day, the questions become when, what, and how much. You eliminate this perilous question: "Should I exercise today?" You can skip that question and be active against cancer.

I do know how hard cancer treatment can be. I'm not advocating that you workout if you are too ill, run-down, or plagued with side effects of treatment that can't be overcome. Chapter ten details how to adjust your exercise schedule during cancer treatment.

FOR HOW LONG?

How long should you walk or do your choice of activity? Ten or twenty minutes are both good starting time periods, depending on your conditioning and your health concerns. Pick a starting duration that seems right to you. These periods are long enough to seem worth the effort and short enough to not be intimidating.

Can you only imagine walking for 5 minutes? Then choose to be active 5 minutes per day. If even that seems unmanageable, walk for half that long, two times per day. At first, you might feel silly, but after a week, you can switch to 5-minute walks and then you're on track.

If you have some residual fitness or feel up to it, start with 20 minutes per session. I don't recommend starting with more than 20 minutes if you are truly starting to exercise after a lay-off, injury, illness, or are receiving cancer treatment.

Isn't more exercise always better? You might think so, but I would disagree. For Starting Plan members, success and continuing to exercise is much more important than the number of minutes involved. You are building a habit of exercise, and to do that, you must keep doing it nearly every day. Stick with it. You are building a foundation for your future health.

In contrast, if you just try to jump to 30 minutes immediately, you may be overwhelmed, become too tired, or become lame. Your reactions could cause you to quit your exercise plan. Instead, try the incremental approach. Start with 10 or 20 minutes and then build up, as described below.

Building Up to Thirty Minutes

After exercising for three weeks at your starting level, add 5 to 10 minutes per day for two weeks. Then add another 5 to 10 minutes for two weeks, if needed, in the same pattern, until you reach 30 minutes per day. Add the new minutes in the amount that seems right to you, depending on your baseline fitness and your comfort. The incremental approach to increasing your duration of exercise will probably seem to be going rather slow, at times, but it will ensure that your body adapts. If it feels right to you, add the minutes faster. You can increase every week instead of every two weeks, for example. The main point is to add minutes in a way that is comfortable. There's nothing wrong with patience as you adapt. Keep the goal time of 30 minutes in mind. You'll get there soon!

Keep track of your progress in written notes. You should be able to progress smoothly, but if you need to make any adjustments, just do so. If you feel that you have good residual strength and conditioning, you can increase from 20 to 30 minutes after three weeks if you want to try it. If it doesn't feel right, adjust accordingly.

HOW FAST?

Do aerobic activity at a pace that seems right to you. Make an effort to exercise comfortably, in a relaxed and focused manner. There are no bonus points for trying to tire yourself out with a speedy pace. Because you are just getting started exercising after a lay-off, illness, surgery, cancer treatment, or an inactive lifestyle, your participation is more important than your pace.

You will elevate your heart rate adequately if you just try to walk slightly faster than a stroll. Focus on your walking. You should be able to talk comfortably and not be out of breath. You don't need to look like a race walker to be benefiting.

Going at a modest speed, rather than trying too hard for a higher intensity, benefits your heart's conditioning. It is common for people to believe that they have to always "push, push, push" if they are doing exercise. Wrong, wrong, wrong! You can focus on staying relaxed and still make progress. I promise.

If you need to slow down, slow down. For example, if you are very tired, generally, but you feel like you are okay to walk, go ahead. Slow down your pace. It is better to do a slow walk than none at all, as long as you can do so safely. A short walk boosts your mood. You will be glad that you didn't just skip it.

If you would like to, add ski poles and do Nordic walking, which is the fancy name for walking with poles. It adds some upper body intensity, helps with balance, and makes a short walk more effortful—and perhaps more fun. It's great on trails. Just adapt a set of ski poles by adding a pair of rubber tips to the ends.

YOUR FLEXIBILITY WORKOUT

To improve flexibility, the simplest route is to take a yoga class once per week. You may want to do your yoga on your day off from aerobic activity. If you are homebound or prefer to do yoga at home, follow along with a yoga video once per week. You can also easily see your progress as you continue with it over time.

Why try yoga for stretching? Yoga instruction is widely available, and you can probably find a class that suits you. Yoga is soothing, pleasant, and can be adapted to your condition. Stretching has not captured the public's imagination, but yoga, with its many benefits, does. It seems as if yoga is everywhere now.

Yoga is actually much more than just stretching. You can receive great benefits for your physical well-being and in terms of stress reduction, along with emotional and mental satisfaction.

Yoga positions, known as poses or postures, all have names. Only some of the yoga poses are complicated, difficult, or intimidating. Yoga may seem intimidating to beginners if they imagine they need to become a human pretzel to succeed at it. You don't have to do complex, strenuous poses at first or, truthfully, ever. As a beginner, you can get a great benefit from some fairly simple and basic positions. You can even adapt these poses to be used if you are sitting or in bed.

One good way to become familiar with the poses is to look at a yoga book with photos of different yoga poses. There is also a yoga deck of cards with poses on each one. I like using those cards to make a sequence of poses for myself. I'm the kind of person who finds it difficult to always follow along with a video or a class. I like to do what feels good in the moment.

You can join classes at a yoga center and learn experientially from an accomplished teacher. Be sure to find a good teacher whose class is not too strenuous or stress-producing for you. The yoga class environment should ideally be supportive emotionally. Don't be intimidated: if the class makes you feel like you will get injured, find a different class.

If you want to do yoga at home, look for a good video at your bookstore, at a bargain store, or online. Gaiam's yoga DVDs are excellent. *Yoga for Beginners*, by Rodney Yee, is an excellent choice. Gaiam's videos are returnable, even if opened, so if for some reason you don't like them, you can get your money back.

A yoga mat helps with keeping your feet in place because the mat is sticky. The mat also provides some padding when you lie on it. Yoga mats can be found online, in some discount chain stores, and in specialty shops.

You'll want to wear loose pants and a stretchy shirt. Buy yoga clothes if you like, but don't feel obligated to be fashion-conscious. Stretchy athletic clothing and yoga-styled clothes are popular and you should be able to find them at all price points.

Some communities have special classes for yoga for cancer survivors. These groups can function like support groups as well as yoga classes. Look for one to join or inspire someone to start one in your community. Perhaps you will be the ideal catalyst for a supportive yoga program that will help others.

Maybe you think that you're not the yoga type. Increasing your flexibility might not seem like exercise to you. It's easy to imagine that it's not very important, compared to being strong and well conditioned aerobically. Why should you care about flexibility?

Flexibility helps you in all your other exercise efforts. It can help prevent injury, keep you youthful, and help your posture. Allowing your muscles to relax, getting familiar with releasing unnecessary tension, and quieting the mind are just some of the great benefits of yoga. Your progress with flexibility will become obvious over time, and if you stick with a yoga practice, you will see many benefits.

In the discussion in chapter twelve, there is more detail about yoga's other important benefits to your well-being. You can also read about yoga in the magazine *Yoga Journal* or on websites. See the resource section of this book.

YOUR STRENGTH PLAN

For your strength training, the best frequency is every other day, three times a week. However, for the purpose of getting you started, you should do the strength training one time each week. With this approach, you can ease into it.

For your strength plan, you should find a program that you actually enjoy and will do regularly. There are many choices and that's good because people have many different tastes in strength-training menus. You might want to use resistance bands, hand weights, weight machines, strength-based yoga or Pilates moves, calisthenics, a medicine ball, or other activities. Carrying firewood or working in the garden also counts.

You might have to try a couple of different approaches before you find one you like, or you may have to change your strategy from time to time to prevent boredom. Or maybe that's just me? First, let's look at a simple home-based program. Then we'll go over some other options.

At-home Simple Strength Plan

For this at-home simple strength plan, you will need ample space for moving and a pair of hand-held weights. Your weights should be somewhere between one pound and ten pounds. The weight should be light enough so that you can do ten repetitions of a move. You may want a variety of weights, in pairs, such as two, five and ten pounds. You will probably need different weights for different exercises.

The first five exercises are for the legs and core muscles. The last four are for the upper body.

1. Squats. Do ten squats, lowering yourself as if you are going to sit in a chair and then rising up again. If this is too challenging, don't lower yourself as far or hold onto something for balance as you do it. To increase the challenge, hold hand-weights as you do the exercise.

2. Wall sits. Stand near a wall and lower yourself, inching your feet forward about 15 inches and reaching a seated-type position with your back against the wall. Hold the position for thirty seconds. To modify this, do not go as low or hold the position as long.

3. Standing one-legged modified squat. Standing on one leg with or without holding onto something for balance, lower your torso while your knee bends forward. Then rise up. Do this ten times. You do not need to go any lower than is comfortable.

4. Lunges. Lunge forward by stepping far forward onto one leg whose knee you bend to about a right angle. Keep your torso upright. Come back to the start position, switch legs, and repeat. Do this ten times. Hold hand-weights to increase the difficulty.

5. Abdominal crunches or yoga's plank (or modified plank) pose. Abdominal crunches can be very effective. Do a number that tires you slightly. You do need not lift your torso up all the way to your bent knees, just enough to engage your core muscles. Or you can do a plank pose, which is like the start of a push-up where your arms are extended straight, but you just hold your torso steady with no lowering. To modify the position and rest your wrists, hold yourself up on your forearms and knees, instead.

6. Push-ups or modified push-ups. Everyone recognizes a push-up. If you can, do ten of them. If you can't, modify it by leaning from a standing position so that you are doing a push-up against your kitchen counter or a wall. The intensity can vary based on how much of your body

weight you are supporting. You can adjust the angle when you get stronger.

7. "Downward-facing dog" yoga pose. If you are able, find an illustration of this pose. Basically, you are supporting the weight of your body on your arms and legs, with your hips being the point of the inverted "V" shape that you make with your body. Hold it for 20 to 30 seconds, breathing in a relaxed manner.

8. Bicep curls. Familiar to most people, a biceps curl can be done with a hand weight that you hold at your side in one hand. Then you lift your hand towards your shoulder, by bending at your elbow. Do ten of these.

9. Triceps curls. Lean forward from the waist and hold onto the back of a chair with one hand, so that your back is parallel is to the floor. Hold a hand weight in your free arm. Keep your feet secure on the floor. No slipping! Now, lift the hand-weight up to your ribs, and then lower it gently and slowly. Do ten of these.

Circuit Training at the Gym

Circuit training simply means that you go from one piece of equipment to another in a sort of circle or circuit, doing work on each piece and ultimately getting a whole-body workout. For this kind of work, you need to be at a gym. You should get personalized instruction on the machines that you will use, whether Nautilus or other circuit machines. Your goal is to develop a routine that is balanced in how it strengthens your whole body.

Many people enjoy going to a gym for weight work because of a gym's social aspects. If you are unfamiliar with going to a gym to lift weights, ask a friend to go with you, or make an appointment with personnel at the gym who can teach you the basics. Some fitness centers have "women only" workout rooms, which can reduce any sense of intimidation.

Using Resistance Bands

Stretchable, plastic, resistance bands, such as Therabands®, can give you new home-based options. You can get instruction from a variety of places. A physical therapist can instruct you on a program to suit your needs, or a personal trainer may help. You can look for DVDs that relate to resistance bands, search for YouTube videos, or look at illustrations in magazine articles.

Using resistance bands is convenient, inexpensive, and easy to do at home. You can tailor the level of difficulty to your needs, by changing the strength of the bands or the length that you stretch. You can work out all the major muscle groups with resistance bands, and they are easily portable if you travel.

DVD-based Strength Programs

Many times it is easiest to workout at home with a DVD for instruction. You might want to look at a website such as Gaiam. com. If you search that site using the key word "strength," you can look at some of their popular DVDs and kits with equipment. Some programs use strategies with resistance bands, balance ball, and hand-weight use. Additional strength workouts are inter-mixed with dance or aerobic workouts.

Another very reliable source of good information is *Prevention* magazine. You can find this at your local library or at a store. The advantage of looking at your library is the chance to review several issues. You are sure to find a few generalized workouts with photos and accurate descriptions. *Prevention*, via Rodale, also has a line of DVDs.

Yoga or Pilates for Strength Training

You can do strengthening as part of your yoga session, if you choose yoga positions that use your body's mass as the weight. Rodney Yee and many other instructors have special programs that are well designed for a strength focus. Alternatively, do a yoga program that has a mix of more gentle poses with strengthening ones. You don't have to do strength work in isolation from stretching if you don't want to.

Alternatively, a Pilates workout can focus on strengthening, in combination with flexibility work. Some people really enjoy Pilates because there is more movement, generally, than in yoga. It is best to take a few classes in person or work one-on-one with an instructor before trying Pilates based on self-instruction and a DVD. Pilates moves require you to have proper core stabilization. If you use improper form, then you risk injuring your back. My physical therapist reports that she sees people injured that way. After some instruction, an at-home workout may be convenient or you may find that a structured class offers support and commitment that help you succeed.

Calisthenics

You can use old-fashioned calisthenics, which are exercises that use your own body weight, including squats, lunges and push-ups. You can put together your own program using this type of exercise. Some DVDs specialize in these old-fashioned, yet effective, moves.

Cross-fit is a relative newcomer on the fitness scene. Cross-fit is a very popular form of using your own body weight, primarily, as a way to do strengthening exercises. In a sequence that changes frequently, a Cross-fit workout takes about 45 minutes to one hour and provides strengthening that can help you do other athletic activities with a better base of strength and more stamina. Look for a program in a gym near you or find more information online.

One cancer survivor whom I interviewed, June, spoke very highly of Cross-fit as a way to regain strength and stamina for her sports. She was weakened by chemotherapy and by her relatively low activity levels that followed. An active person, by nature, who likes skiing, golf and other sports, June needed a way to recover her stamina for those activities after her first phase of treatment ended. She found Cross-fit very helpful in regaining fitness and strength. It became like a sport in itself to her. June looks forward to her sessions as a stress reliever and an enjoyable workout. Her cancer recovery is going well, and she even scored her best ever round of golf while in chemotherapy.

Choosing Your Strength-training Activities

Your goal, in the long run is to find what works for you, your lifestyle, your budget, your timeframe, and your sense of what is enjoyable. You should be able to find something that you will do and stick with doing.

How do you decide what to do? The choice involves your current strength, any health concerns, and your taste in activities. You may want to choose your strength routine with the help of a personal trainer, physical therapist, or friend. A customized program may help you make good progress and prevent any injuries. If all else fails, use trial and error until some type of program sticks!

Are you worried about bulking up too much? Some women do worry about gaining weight or size because they are lifting weights or doing other strength work. You probably don't need to worry. Most people who gain more strength will lose fat and gain muscle. You won't bulk up significantly unless you lift heavy weights. Don't worry if early strengthening work doesn't equate with pounds lost; if you're trading fat for muscle, it's all to the good.

Gaining muscle mass has the advantage of helping you to raise your base metabolism, which is the rate at which your body converts fuel to energy. You will burn more calories at rest than you would with less muscle. Having adequate strength and muscle mass can also help fight osteoporosis, diabetes, and heart disease. Additionally, being stronger will help open up the door to enjoying your exercise more and more.

SUMMARY

Our resident skeptic might ask: "Is a good exercise plan really this simple?" Yes! If you combine an aerobic element with some stretching and some strengthening, you are well underway. You're soon ahead of most people because you will be in the habit of exercising daily. After you have the habit of daily exercise, you can move onto activities that are more interesting to you.

If you have special health concerns that make the Starting Plan too difficult, go directly to chapter ten now and read about how to adjust this plan to your needs. You should find some alternatives that will work for you. Remember, check with your doctor first. And if you have any questions, get personalized, professional advice.

Do you have time now to lace up your shoes and go for a walk? Here is the absolute best trick that I know for getting out the door if you are de-motivated. Get in your appropriate clothes and put on your appropriate shoes. Tell yourself that you don't "have to" go for a walk at all. Then, go stroll around your yard a minute or two. See what happens next! Excuses are so flimsy. They will disappear when you're out the door ready to go. So... have a nice walk!.

❋ ❋ ❋

ACTIVE SURVIVOR PROFILE: DENISE

DOING WHAT SHE CAN TO STAY HEALTHY

One day when Denise was at the local bagel shop, still wearing her purple doo-rag to cover her chemo-bald head, a woman approached her and said, "You rock. You are my idol."

Puzzled, Denise waited for an explanation. The woman continued, "I see you at the gym all the time, working out, even though you are obviously going through cancer treatment. I figure if you can be there working out, then what's my excuse? I can workout, too."

Denise continued with regular exercise throughout her two cancer bouts and her treatment periods. She says, "I just kept doing it. Exercise helps my well-being, boosts my endorphins, and gives me great satisfaction. I am not a happy camper if I can't exercise."

Denise's first breast cancer experience included a lumpectomy and radiation treatments. She had always exercised before cancer, so she kept up with it during her treatment. Although she didn't get specific guidance, her treatment team was supportive of her continuing physical exercise. The radiation oncologist helped her figure out how to protect her skin. She used a product called Aqua Seal on her skin so that she could swim.

Denise continued regular workouts at the gym three times a week: she would ride the exercise bike, do her weight training, and then swim. She emphasized upper body exercise, working the pectoral muscles and doing bench work with five-pound to seven-pound dumbbells. The radiation oncologist remarked that Denise's skin stayed very healthy during the process, which Denise attributes to the exercise keeping the blood flowing to the irradiated area. The muscles, also, didn't get "clamped down" and the muscle structure "didn't stiffen" she said.

Denise's second bout with breast cancer was more complex: she had two mastectomies and chemotherapy. Again, Denise kept exercising. She rode her bike or walked for exercise while she healed from the surgery. When she was allowed, Denise increased her upper body exercise. She received lymph massage to improve circulation to the chest. Denise had "zero issues with lymphedema." She chose not to get reconstructive surgery and wears only a sports bra for compression, rather than any special compression garments.

During her chemotherapy, Denise followed a pattern: she received chemotherapy on Thursday, did not feel great Friday and Saturday, but she went back to the gym on Monday. She had four treatments, three weeks apart. When her blood counts lowered, she slowed down. As a biology instructor, Denise knows her physiology. Knowing that leg exercise takes more oxygen than upper-body work, she cut back on her leg exercises. At one point, she had an eye infection and was hospitalized because her white blood cell counts were so low. However, in general, she says, even though her blood counts went down periodically, "my numbers always came right back up."

With the first bout with breast cancer, Denise continued working. During the second bout, she took a leave of absence from her job. She made sure to listen to her body and get adequate rest. Denise also began to work with a personal trainer, who had her do circuit training with an emphasis on martial arts.

Denise credits exercise with helping her to eat better, stimulating her appetite, and helping her drink more fluids. Because she went to a gym when her white blood counts were low, she tried to pick times when the gym wasn't especially busy. She also used hand sanitizer to alleviate the risk of infection. She felt comfortable with her levels of risk.

Talking philosophically, Denise says that "going through cancer made me realize not to take good health for granted. I can't control if I get something else—I had melanoma last winter—but I can control what I eat and how much I exercise. I do whatever I can to stay healthy." Meanwhile, with her strong attitude and consistent efforts to take care of herself, Denise also became a role model to her daughter, her trainer, her doctors, her nurses, and apparently, strangers at the gym. She rocked!

CHAPTER EIGHT

SUSTAINING PLAN: OPTIMAL ACTIVITIES FOR CANCER RECOVERY

I n the Sustaining Plan, your goals are to build up your fitness, strength and flexibility with a steady program of physical activities. This plan will help you sustain your exercise habit and can help you sustain your health. You will spend more time being active, using the same good habits that you have already developed. Based on the American College of Sports Medicine's recommendations for cancer survivors, you will keep getting a minimum of 30 minutes of aerobic exercise five times per week, plus do strengthening and flexibility work.

As mentioned previously, this plan is appropriate for during cancer treatment as well as after treatment ends. In the next chapter, there is extensive discussion of adjustments that you can make to this plan when the need arises.

SUSTAINING PLAN SUMMARY

- Do 30 minutes of aerobic training five times per week.

- Do strength training one to three times per week.

- Do one hour to 90 minutes of yoga per week.

- Optional: Start to use either an easy or faster pace during workouts. Do an easy pace one day and a faster pace the next day, repeating this pattern.

- Optional: Substitute other aerobic sports and activities for walking to keep up your interest in exercise as needed.

- Optional: Start to do some endurance training by doing 45 to 60 minutes of aerobic activity once each week, or eventually more, if your health allows.

WALKING AS YOUR AEROBIC ACTIVITY CHOICE

For as long as you want, stick with walking as your aerobic activity if it works for you. There are some benefits to continuing to make walking your choice. You can measure your progress easily if you keep to the same activity. Walking is easy to adapt to your needs, if you have any issues with side effects. It's convenient, easy to do, and usually a refreshing way to get outdoors in good weather. Many people take a daily walk as a rewarding, lifelong habit.

PACE

Any aerobic venture should begin at an easy pace for 5 minutes. Call it your warm-up period and make it part of your routine. In a warm-up, you are literally warming up the muscles and getting your heart rate up without over-doing. A good warm-up can mean the difference between an enjoyable session and a frustrating one.

Here's a short physiology lesson about something that might be counter to one's intuition. Do you think starting out a walk really fast would be the most effective way to lose fat? We might think that if we push ourselves, then we must benefit. In reality, physiology says otherwise. There is a more subtle logic to when you should push your pace.

If you immediately start a run, for instance, at a high pace, you start the adrenaline system because the body thinks of it as an emergency and wants to provide all the necessary energy so you can run hard. You don't draw on your fat reserves. If, on the other hand, you start slowly, your slower-burning energy stores can be drawn on and, overall, you will more effectively burn fat. In the same way, starting your walk at an easy pace as a warm-up is ideal. The lesson? Don't push the pace when you start out. Warm-up slowly.

CHANGING PACE: EASY AND FASTER PACES

Each time that you go out for a walk, do your warm-up at a slow pace. Then, on alternate days, do a pace appropriate to either an easy day or faster day.

For your easy day, go at a speed that feels like you could keep up a conversation easily without being out of breath. Another way to describe the pace is to imagine that you would have to go at this speed all day. (Imagine!) This pace is very relaxing. It might take you a while to find out what the speed is, for you, but it will be clear when you find it.

For your faster day, you will speed up your walking compared to the easy pace. How much? Try to go at a pace that is a bit challenging but still comfortable. You might breathe more intentionally, but you won't feel breathless. You can comfortably talk in short phrases, however, you might talk less than before. Your heart rate will be more elevated, but it won't pound through your chest. This faster-day pace is not the fastest that you can go. It's not like race walking. Picture, instead, walking briskly.

If you are in cancer treatment, you may have all you can manage without worrying about pace changes. If all you can do is to get out and walk at whatever pace comes, that's fine. These alternating pace changes provide you with an option to keep walking interesting. They build up your conditioning levels well. With paces that vary, you will see after some time that your faster pace gets faster, over time, yet stays comfortable. Good job!

STRENGTH TRAINING: EACH WEEK

In the Sustaining Plan, you should do strengthening exercises one to three times a week. The number of sessions is up to you, depending on your goals, your other activities, and your interest in strengthening. You will see the most improvement in strengthening when you do the workouts three times per week, which is widely agreed upon by fitness trainers as the optimum number. However, if your aerobic sports also build strength, you may forego the second and third weekly strength training sessions. Your goal is to have a strength program that challenges you the right amount. When you enjoy your program, you will keep it up. Sometimes having a goal of being strong enough to do more sports activities keeps you on track.

To do strength work three times per week, take a day off in between each session. The days off between strength workouts are critical because they allow your muscles, which get slightly injured during the workout, to have time to heal, recover, and become stronger. Lifting more than you are ready to lift is not recommended.

To determine what type of strength training to do, review the options in the previous chapter. You may do the same things each time you train or perhaps you will like doing a variety of activities. Find personalized advice about your choices if you plan to emphasize strength training, otherwise your workout from the Starting Plan can just be continued. If you have any special medical concerns from your cancer treatment, please make sure your strength workout plans are tailored to you and get professional help if you need it.

Whom should you ask for help personalizing your program? A physical therapist is your best consulting professional if you have some definite physical limitations from injuries or side effects. If your concerns are more focused on your own conditioning quirks, try a personal trainer. You might have, for example, strong legs but weak arms. Or you might have a weak core and not know how to address it with exercise. Tell your consultant about your cancer history. If they want more information about oncology-related questions, they should be able to contact the ACSM or your doctor.

FLEXIBILITY: AN HOUR OF YOGA EACH WEEK

Keep going with the yoga that you began doing in the Starting Plan. You didn't start yoga yet? Add it now. Review the yoga sections in previous chapter. As your yoga experience grows, you will probably get more and more out of it. Enjoy the subtle beauty of the yoga experience, and savor the present moment.

BUILDING ENDURANCE

The ACSM's *Exercise Guidelines for Cancer Survivors* call for five 30-minute periods of aerobic activity each week. That is a sufficient amount of time for most people in cancer treatment or early cancer recovery. Please stay with that amount if you are in a health crisis.

On the other hand, if your overall health is now good and your side effects of treatment have resolved sufficiently, you may want to expand one of the 30-minute periods to 45-minutes to make more fitness gains.

If you are up to lengthening your workout, try to add 15 minutes this way: lengthen your easy warm-up period to 10 minutes, then walk more briskly for 30 minutes, then cool down for 5 minutes. This lengthening of your exercise time period should not be appreciably hard if you have no other medical issues at this time.

You might really enjoy spending longer being active, doing something recreational, and relaxing. It's rejuvenating. Taking 45 minutes to support your health feels really good. The first half hour seems like merely a good start at relaxing. Why would you want to quit when you're starting to relax?

Near the end of this chapter, after the section on activities and sports, I further discuss endurance training. Let me be clear: developing much greater endurance is a good goal for when you are healthy, out of active cancer treatment, and in stable condition. If you are in treatment or early recovery, stick with the once-per-week longer outing for now.

CHOOSING YOUR ACTIVITIES AND SPORTS

Everyone likes different sports. After a while, you may get bored with walking and want to find another activity to enjoy. As you know, there are many choices. You can look for the type of exercise that makes you happy from among an endless number of choices. It's great to learn some new sports activity and be a beginner again. There really is something for everyone, whether you like speed or you avoid it, whether you like a lot of sweating or being in the pool, whether you like to paddle on calm lakes or whitewater. If you haven't found your niche in sports, please keep looking.

I'm a cross-country skier who likes the graceful, repetitious motions of that sport. I like being outdoors in winter and skiing uphill. My husband is a downhill racer. He makes big arcing turns most of the time. He likes to tuck and go fast in a race-course. We're different, but we favor our own particular brand of skiing fun. You have to find what you love to do. By the way, don't worry about us: sometimes we ski together.

Here is a short summary of some of the features of popular individual aerobic sports, with highlights of their rewards.

Bicycling

Bicycling is great for beginners and for people who don't enjoy impact activities. Riding a bike can be, well, as easy as riding a bike. One of the best summaries of how to get in shape was, in my opinion, written in a tweet by Lance Armstrong. I don't know his exact words, but his advice to someone who wanted to get fit was something like this: Get a bike, ride it every day, eat right, and get enough rest. That's really a great summation of the crucial advice.

One of the reasons top athletes reach their goals is because they make things very simple. Get a bike, ride it every day, eat right, and get enough rest. Everything else is a matter of details, whether your goal is the podium in Paris or making health gains for the sake of fighting cancer.

For bike riding, all you need is a bike, a well-fitting helmet, and stiff-soled, comfortable shoes. They don't have to be bike shoes, at first. Many cyclists get very involved with their gear choices and expensive biking clothes, but I remember riding every day for a month in two-dollar gym shorts and five-dollar sneakers and being no worse for it. Of course, life was simpler in 1981. No matter. If you have a modest budget, go to a bike swap sale or look for end-of-year deals. Get a bargain on a decent bike and ride it wearing whatever clothes you have. The right bright-colored, high-tech clothes, special bike shoes, and top-notch bike gear are excellent. Just don't think you can't ride an old junker sometimes. If you have a helmet and a bike, you're ready to start.

Make some friends who also ride and join up with groups based in your community. You don't have to compete in races to join a bike club. Just have fun and enjoy long bike rides with company. Competitive cycling includes something for everyone: mountain biking, club events, riding as part of a fundraiser, or in a triathlon. You can also enjoy scenic trail rides on designated bike paths or long tours for the tourist with pedal power. You can take slow Sunday jaunts in your neighborhood. Bike camping is also a possibility.

Are you timid about riding on the skinny tires of racing bikes, but you still want to ride a bike? Try a cross bike that combines features of mountain bikes with a design more suited for roads or level paths. You can ride on dirt roads that have less traffic with a cross bike or mountain bike, or you can find recreational trails, such as rails-to-trails, that are not open to cars. Don't forsake biking until you consider all options. There are even tandem bikes, if you want to pair up with someone.

Cycling is great for all levels of fitness and especially friendly to people who want to make improvements when starting from scratch. Plus, those downhills are really fun! Start by getting on your bike at least every weekend and build up your skills and fitness.

Running and Trail Running

I love the simplicity of running. When I lace up my shoes for a run, I feel like a kid. I'm about to have an adventure, relax, enjoy the weather and get energized. In my head or aloud, I'm singing and I'm happy. I do realize that not everyone gets that much enjoyment from running, but I just want to tell you that it is possible.

To enjoy running, you may want to work on your technique. An excellent book, *Chi Running* by Danny Dreyer, outlines how to streamline your form so that your running is comfortable, natural and efficient. Don't just plod along with awkward footfalls and bad posture. Please know that even though running is simple, good form is not automatic. You may benefit enormously, right at the start of your running career, by having an expert runner help you with form and technique.

For inspiration, advice, and plenty of how-to articles, go to your library and browse through *Runner's World* or other running magazines. Ask for help from friends or acquaintances. Runners are very common. There's a high likelihood that you know some runners or can join a local running club. Beginners are welcomed in almost every club.

Trail running is my secret heaven on earth. I love to run among the trees, roots, and rocks of the local woods and fields. Trail running is gentler on my spine, less bruising to my leg muscles, less repetitious in its motions, and very meditative. It provides a more intense experience of the natural surroundings. I feel like a wild, free animal. Even when I am running slowly, my senses feel alive and full of pleasure. Plus, I can always stop to rest, listen for birds, and enjoy a meditative moment.

Switch from Walking to Running

If you have progressed with your walking program to 30-minute walks, would you like to try running? Make the transition gradually and it should go well.

There are many considerations for new runners, such as getting good running shoes, avoiding early injuries from overuse, and developing good body mechanics for running. (Hint: Don't run with bad posture, extra tension, awkward gait, or bad foot placement. Read Danny Dreyer's important book *Chi Running* for perfectly clear, well-illustrated advice.) Ideally, you should work with someone like a personal trainer, avid runner, or physical therapist that can help you avoid any rookie mistakes. Alternatively, you can ask local running club members their advice. Sometimes you'll find a program made for people like you or a mentor in a club.

How to Advance to Running for Thirty Minutes

Here's a program to get you started running. The basic idea is to add running, in small amounts, to your walk over weeks. You will gradually increase the time spent running. This program is the type recommended to runners coming back from injuries. If the program seems to progress too quickly for you, as a new runner, repeat each week's variation for two weeks, instead of just one. On the days off, continue your walking program. Donna Smyers, athlete and physical therapist, wrote this program.

- Week One. Warm up with 5 minutes of walking before you add the running segments. During a 30-minute walk, add eight intervals of one minute of running. Separate the running intervals by 2 minutes of walking this week and on each of the future weeks.

- Week Two. After you warm up, as above, add 5 intervals of 2 minutes of running. Separate the running intervals with 2 minutes of walking.

- Week Three. Add 3 intervals of 4 minutes.

- Week Four. Add 3 intervals of 6 minutes.

- Week Five. Add 3 intervals of 8 minutes.

- After a 5-minute warm-up, run 20 minutes, and cool down with 5 minutes of walking.

This program worked well for me after a six-month lay-off caused by a complex knee injury and ACL knee surgery. The progression called for some patience and some faith, but it was pain-free and very effective. If you have any pain when starting to run, do seek help from a physical therapist or other professional. An ounce of prevention is worth a pound of cure.

Swimming

No sport is more gentle on your body than swimming. Swimming also provides an aerobic challenge and helps your fitness. Pools are widely available, and fresh water swimming is available many places, at least seasonally. If you are a non-swimmer, take a class for beginners. Most people can learn to swim and being able to enjoy swimming is a pleasure.

If you are a mediocre swimmer, you might enjoy the sport more if you improved your technique. Like most aerobic sports, the key is to use efficient effective motions to accomplish forward movement without wasting much effort. Get individualized coaching on technique from other swimmers or swim instructors. You will be thrilled if you swim more easily and efficiently.

Many excellent swimmers will take short rests during their swim times. In a pool, it is easy to fashion a workout where you swim a lap, rest 5 or 10 seconds, swim farther, and repeat. You can adjust the length of time that you spend swimming to create patterns called pyramids. These structures help the yards—and the time—go by more quickly.

There is just something about a good swim that makes your body feel wonderful. How beautifully refreshing it is to swim in cool water in the hot summer weather. Or you can escape bad outdoor weather with a trip to the local pool. As a bonus, swimming is a great way to burn calories, has no impact, and is a great weight-loss strategy.

Cross-country Skiing

Do you live where winters are long and cold? Do you notice that people who ski or snowshoe seem happy when it snows? Nordic skiing is my favorite sport. I can't even estimate how much fitness—and pleasure—I have derived from cross-country skiing.

For years, I taught beginners to ski. In 90 minutes, most people can learn to cross-country ski with grace and efficiency. One simple lesson can lead to a lifelong enjoyment of skiing. Don't avoid instruction or you risk developing ineffective technique that is more like walking on skis. Skiing well is only hard if you practice skiing poorly over and over. You will be greatly rewarded for a forward lean in your torso, perfect timing, a longer glide phase, and stronger kick. Get some rhythmic ease and power into your cross-country skiing. Don't settle for trudging along or you'll miss the fun.

Cross-country skiing is a wonderful life-long sport for several reasons. First, there is no impact on the spine because your feet are always on the ground. Second, it strengthens and tones every muscle of the body, including the ever-important core muscles. Skiing also burns a lot of calories per hour. It is easy to adjust how far you want to ski, how fast, or how hard. Last, cross-country takes you outdoors in winter comfortably. The skiing effort keeps you warm and twenty-degree weather feels ideal when you are skiing along. What a way to be active in winter!

Using Exercise Machines

If you look around at most gyms, you will see these exercise machines: rowers, elliptical trainers, bikes (several kinds), and treadmills. You can use any of these for your 30-minute aerobic workouts. If you want to mix it up, you can also try doing 10 minutes on each of three different kinds of equipment. I enjoy that combination because, otherwise, I tend to get bored using exercise machines.

If you're going to workout at a fitness center, ask for some help getting started on unfamiliar equipment. Someone should be available to show you how to run the electronics and how to use the equipment safely. People are usually glad to help, as long as you are not interrupting their workout at a bad time.

One advantage of using gym equipment is that you can easily test your pulse rate on many machines. Then, you can learn more about your optimal workout heart rate zones. Get help from a personal trainer or other fitness professional to tailor your workouts according to your heart-rate zones.

Fun Activity Classes to Try

While you are at the fitness club, you could also try Zumba classes or other dance classes. Ballroom dancing, swing dancing, and other dance activities, in classes or socially, are also great activities if you favor exercising gracefully to music. In the New York City area, check out "Moving On Aerobics," an innovative, well-researched dance aerobics program that supports people who are healing from cancer.

Maybe you can join a water aerobics class. Hint: Water aerobics is great for people who want a fun, effective workout with no impact. Being in the water also feels like playing and the workouts seem easy, although they provide good exercise. Water aerobics won't help you build bone mass, however, because of the lack of impact, so do some walking for bone strength, as well.

Other Sports

There is a long list of sports that you can enjoy: golf, tennis, racquetball, bowling, ice skating, soccer, lacrosse, basketball, snowshoeing, and ultimate Frisbee. From horseback riding to triathlons, each sport will have its devotees. From the outside as a novice, it can look difficult to advance in a new sport. We each have our own tolerances for new experiences, but if you're a cancer survivor, you might have a fresh openness to trying new things. Consider fulfilling an old dream or taking up a new active hobby or lifestyle. Follow your interests and enjoy.

MORE ENDURANCE TRAINING: AN EVENTUAL GOAL?

The ACSM has guidelines not only for cancer survivors, but also for all the population. In these broader, general guidelines, as I have mentioned, the ACSM states that a routine workout period of 45 to 60 minutes, five days each week, is preferable for people who can achieve it. Health benefits accrue from the increased fitness and strength.

After doing longer time periods of exercise, you will see that improvements to your conditioning, strength and performance come more easily. With more endurance, you can enjoy your favorite activities for longer periods. To me, that equals having more fun in life. Many sports, such as bike riding or cross-country skiing, do lend themselves well to longer outings.

Don't take on significant endurance training during active cancer treatment or too early in your recovery, especially if it is new to you. However, after you are returned to good health, and if you have kept up with your exercise routine, you can start to do longer periods of exercise more frequently than once per week.

To build up endurance, go longer and go slower. Whatever your fitness level is, when you want to expand your endurance, you simply go farther and go as slowly as you need to. Being continuously active for over 45 minutes helps your cardiovascular conditioning and builds up your ability to enjoy longer periods of exercise.

It is best to add time to your usual daily aerobic exercise periods, incrementally and systematically. You can add 10 minutes to a daily workout each week, usually, with no problems. Some athletes will designate one workout per week as their over-distance or very long time period, inching that one up by increments of ten to fifteen minutes weekly. Eventually, if you have one day each week with an hour to two hours of aerobic exercise, you will find that you have gained a lot of fitness. Remember, the lower the intensity of your effort, the longer you can be active. You can judge subjectively or with heart-rate watches, which are now easy to use and affordable. For more information on training by understanding your heart rate information, see Stu Mittleman's book *Slow Burn: Burn Fat Faster by Exercising Slower*. His advice is superb for beginners through experts, whom he helps train for faster racing.

When you are ready to add longer periods of exercise, your enthusiasm can get ahead of your fitness. Don't get hurt overdoing it. Increase your exercise volume slowly and steadily. If you do too much and get lame, you are likely to get discouraged. On the other hand, the slower that you go, the farther you can go. Runners can extend their workouts by walking for intervals of time, and walkers can extend their workouts by walking more slowly. Enjoy being active longer!

If you are primarily walking for your aerobic fitness, adding a longer hike once per week is a lovely way to make gains. When hiking, you can rest as much as you need to. Your motivation can benefit by having a goal of a summit view or by making the outing a social one. Hiking is a great path to fitness and strength accessible to many people.

I feel the positive effects of a longer workout period for hours after I stop moving. That positive, energized sense of vitality is why a lot of runners and others like to workout for long periods. It feels so good, both during and after. For many athletes, their exercise is their daily mood-lifter and their stress-buster. After you start to see how great you can feel after a moderately long walk, you may get hooked, yourself.

For more tips on endurance conditioning, you can seek out books, magazines, online resources, or coaching from your local sports club. The Team-in-Training program, which is described in chapter fourteen, includes an online coaching feature that can help you to become an endurance athlete in one of several sports. Your best resource may be the people who are already doing what you want to do. Sometimes, all you need to do is start asking around in the network of people that you know.

EXERCISE IN BALANCE WITH REST AND SLEEP

This section discusses the important topic of rest and sleep, which may come up for you at any time. Some people—and you know who you are—become so involved with exercise that they actually deny themselves enough rest or enough sleep. However, most athletic people learn that exercise has to be balanced with getting enough rest and sleep. You simply can't run yourself ragged with sports and expect good results. Finding the right balance is crucial.

The need for balance is doubly relevant for cancer patients. People who are in cancer treatment have some pretty unusual health challenges, and getting adequate rest is very important. Here are some questions that can help you.

1. Am I getting enough exercise to help my health?

2. Am I getting enough rest for my medical and personal needs?

3. Am I getting enough sleep?

You shouldn't use exercise in a way that is exhausting or deleterious to your health. Luckily, it will be pretty easy to judge if you are getting a balance of exercise and rest. Just pay attention to how you feel. Ideally, the dose of exercise that you choose will lift your energy level.

There are two other places in this book to look for information about fatigue, which is well covered because it is so important. Look in chapter ten for a variety of ways to adjust your exercise plans when you are tired. Look in chapter eleven under the subheading "Fatigue" for a general discussion. If you still have questions about how to get the right amount of rest, talk with a sports trainer, physical therapist, or your doctor. Don't exhaust yourself. That's a negative for your cancer recovery. Your goal is good health; do rest adequately.

❋ ❋ ❋

ACTIVE SURVIVOR PROFILE: RAYMOND

COMMITMENT TO EXERCISE

Raymond Hayes was coping with the after-effects of surgery for colon cancer and the early months of a chemotherapy regimen. He was coping, but he was also suffering from nausea related to his 48-hour infusion of Folfox. His white blood cell count was down, which resulted in a sense of constant fatigue. Raymond was going through the motions of his daily life, but he felt too poorly to make it to the gym to exercise. In order to help relieve his nausea, Raymond's medical team suggested switching him to a different anti-nausea medication.

The new drug worked well, and his nausea relented enough for him to be more active. Raymond adopted a strategy that he would follow for the rest of his six months of chemo. His twice-monthly infusion lasted from Wednesday through Friday. Afterward, he would rest up on Saturday and Sunday, and then

Raymond would go back to work Monday. This schedule left him able to go to the office's fitness gym about five days of each two-week period.

When Raymond was able to go to the gym and be more active, he saw his blood counts improve, even as his chemotherapy's other side effects continued. Raymond believed that his exercise was helping him, so in his words, he "forced himself" to exercise. He thought of his exercise commitment as a test of his willpower. The benefits of regular exercise, Raymond thought, were partly physical and partly mental. He believed that the exercise helped "reactivate" his digestive system and "get everything going," including his appetite, digestive processes, and his thirst. He knew that he should force fluids after chemotherapy infusions. When he worked out at the gym, he wanted to drink more water spontaneously, which was much easier than forcing fluids if he was inactive.

Raymond's program at the gym had a balance of activities: he included strength training and aerobic exercise as well as stretching. He lifted weights, rode the stationary bike, and did core strengthening exercises after he received the go-ahead six weeks post-surgery.

Because the gym that Raymond used was at his workplace, he would see colleagues. Most of them knew that he was going through cancer treatment and sympathized. It offered a certain level of social support when people asked after his health and chatted with him at the gym. The exercise itself also provided a morale boost.

In Raymond's words: "My world was shattered; nothing was the same. I continued to work as best I could which was about 60 to 70 percent of the time. As a single, active person, staying home alone felt like a self-imposed prison. Going to the gym at least felt normal. It was encouraging knowing that my infrequent visits were enough to prevent all my muscle mass from disintegrating. My spirits always felt improved just being there."

At home, Raymond walked his dog every day, partly in loyalty to his dog's well being and partly to prove to himself that he was still okay enough to do so. One of the side effects of his chemo treatment was extreme sensitivity to cold temperatures. It was a cold winter in his Pennsylvania town that year, which made being outside difficult. He had to bundle up to protect himself from the cold. As he put on all his layers to go for a walk, Raymond felt like an astronaut preparing himself.

Raymond says that he did think about Lance Armstrong from time to time. He wore Livestrong shirts to the gym. He thought of it as his armor, and felt connected to other cancer survivors. Ray went to the gym even if he felt lethargic beforehand, telling himself that exercise was worth doing.

Raymond, who had completed half-marathon running races in the past, says he no longer feels the need to try a marathon. Cancer treatment survival felt like an endurance race to him, he said, about six months after he finished treatment. He does look forward to get back to doing his regular sports again, but he isn't focused on racing for now.

If treatment compares to a race, then Ray appears to have had a strong finish. He completed his treatment regimen without needing any reduction in his optimal chemotherapy doses. To Raymond, that completed series, at first, did not seem terribly remarkable. Then, his doctor told him that 96 percent of similar patients needed dose reductions. In other words, Ray was among the 4 percent who finish the treatment as planned. Raymond was told he has a 90 to 95 percent five-year cancer-free survival chance, compared to only an 80 to 85 percent chance if he had not completed the doses. As a result of that news, Ray remarked that he was really happy that he had stayed so focused on exercising.

When I spoke to Ray in August of 2010, he had just returned from a ski trip to Argentina with friends. He continues to enjoy his workouts and has added some yoga. Unfortunately, he tore a calf muscle in June when he resumed his running–with perhaps too much intensity, he admits. He enjoys some kayaking, and he will be adding more of his favorite activities, such as hiking, mountain biking, and running.

Raymond is continuing to experience some peripheral neuropathy, but his cold sensitivity is gone now. His dog is still getting walked and, this coming winter, Ray expects to ski on the slopes of the Poconos, healthy, happy, and active.

CHAPTER NINE

TIPS FOR SUCCESS WITH EXERCISE

Distilled from a lifetime of recreational sports, here are my top tips for succeeding with exercise. Some of the tips will be very useful to you, perhaps, and other tips might seem obvious. I have presented them in a loosely organized fashion. You can read them out of order, if you like, and take whatever nuggets you find interesting.

DO EVERYTHING: YOUR SELF-CARE CHOICES

Realize that no matter what your background, fitness level, or experience, you can make exercise part of your recovery. You can choose and develop a positive outlook about exercise during your cancer treatment. During a cancer ordeal, you can take control of the meaningful things that you can do to help your health. You can reinvent your beliefs about exercise, if you need to. See Lawrence Leshan's great book, *Cancer as a Turning Point*, for more on how to re-prioritize during your challenging time.

If you want to build a better relationship with your body, you can use cancer recovery as a way to bring your view of your physical state into a positive framework. Can you imagine thinking good things about your body while you are suffering from cancer? Absolutely! It's cancer that you don't like. It's your body, your health, and your life that you are fighting for. Get on the active side of the fight.

Try to set aside any negative body self-image and start to invest in loving your physical self. If you need help, speak to a counselor, a mentor, a psychologist, or a friend who can be a role model. Take advantage of this chance to change.

SET YOUR ROUTINE AND MARK YOUR CALENDAR

The good news: It only takes three weeks to make a habit. Exercise routinely for just three weeks and you will find that you have made a new habit. You can enjoy being active without having to work so hard each time at finding the motivation. When the question is "What time will I do exercise?" instead of "Will I exercise?" then you are on your way to exercise success. The bad news: You might not reach the third week of exercise if you don't plan well.

The first step is to put exercise on your calendar. Put down the times that you will exercise each day. When will you do what? Look at your calendar and be realistic. Where are the gaps in your schedule?

Break the first three weeks down into one-week portions. Some people will like to exercise first thing in the morning to leave their day's structure as it is. Many people like morning workout periods after some practice with getting up earlier. They start their regular day's agenda all charged up and already ahead. Some people can find a lunch-hour activity slot is a great fit for their busy day. It recharges them for the end of the workday. Others choose an end-of-day or evening slot when they can fully decompress.

You can have the same time slot every day or mix it up to suit your needs and those of people who depend on you. The main thing to do is make a clear choice. Try your plan and then adjust it, if it doesn't work well. Even the nation's president and first lady have exercise on their busy schedules. Keep looking at your calendar until you see the openings.

KEEP AN EXERCISE LOG

Keeping an exercise log or journal can be a big help in your efforts to stay on track with exercise. Here is one way to keep a journal. Get a small lined notebook. Write "Exercise Journal" and the start date on the cover. Hey, that looks good already!

On the first page, write your general and specific goals for the next three or four weeks. On another blank page, list the dates of that week with space in between. Here, you can add in your activity goals before you do them. You can write your notes about the experiences afterwards.

My own entries look like this: "Ran 2 mi. with Mo, felt good, dirt roads, hilly." "Over-distance today. Ran/walked 90 minutes. Felt great." I loosely keep track of time spent, intensity and type of activity. My entries during chemotherapy were ever more brief: "swam" or "walked." My times, intensity and speed didn't matter to me during chemotherapy, only the record of actually doing something active.

After fifteen years of mostly keeping notes for each week of athletic activities I did, I can tell you about my experience. First, when I keep a journal, it spurs me on to try to do something every day that is worth writing down. I don't know why it's so effective to just keep track, but I love filling in entries. When I scan over the last few months of entries, I can touch on lots of good memories, see progress, and feel proud of my exercise accomplishments. Just reading last week's entries can help my resolve to exercise the following week. My notes can help me see immediately why my fitness is improving.

Conversely, if I have been skipping some workouts, it becomes obvious when I look at my notes. When I see blank weeks or days, I am forced to be honest with myself that I'm not getting enough exercise. Sometimes I can often shake off the exercise blahs by looking at the notebook and setting some goals for the upcoming months or seasons. Maybe I need more variation in activities, a better venue, or a race to prepare for.

In some ways, getting through your cancer recovery is like coming back from a very complicated injury. (Okay, I know it's different in about a hundred ways, too, but bear with me a minute.) If you have lower stamina, shorter workouts, and less strength during a long period of treatment, you can still make progress. When you look at your exercise journal, you can see that you are getting closer to the end of treatment. As you start to recover strength and fitness, you can record your progress. Just seeing a record of your improvements can help you stay motivated to exercise.

Keeping track of what I have done helps me plan what to do next. If you want to plan, some day, for a certain event, a race, or a long-term goal, you should plan out your workouts in writing and keep track. You might as well start now! When you see your exercise journal's notes filling up page after page, you can be sure that you are making progress. It's fulfilling. I more than recommend keeping an exercise journal. I think keeping a log may be the single most important thing you can do to keep yourself on track.

SMALL STEPS ADD UP TO FITNESS GAINS

Most fitness gains are incremental. Actually, maybe all fitness gains are incremental! It can be hard to see the point of one short outing of walking or one brief bike ride. Initially, you might not see that 15 minutes of walking is contributing towards your being able to run five kilometers. That's the truth, though. Small gains in fitness quickly add up.

During the past year, I received physical therapy for a complex knee injury. I had my ACL rebuilt with surgery. For one stage of my rehab, I had a 5-minute stationary bike ride for my maximum aerobic workout. Five minutes! It seemed so short to me. However, the 5-minute stationary bike ride today became next week's 10-minute ride, then became a 20-minute ride, and so on, until I was strong again. Incremental progress is really all there is! Thinking of it in context, a 5-minute workout sounded great. Especially compared to all those weeks when I couldn't walk at all.

If you are in treatment for cancer, the idea of making 10 minutes of walking important may strike you as strange at first. You are getting life-saving state-of-the-art medical treatment. How can just a small amount of exercise be very important? Small amounts of exercise are valuable in two ways. First, your body likes it. Secondly, though, continuing to exercise is the path to doing more exercise and getting the optimal benefits to your health.

There is no shortcut. Progress comes in small steps. Value those small steps, those 15-minute swims, and those 20-minute bike rides. You can only enjoy great fitness if you have worked your way up to it. Take a step forward and then take another step.

SET SPECIFIC GOALS

Because it can be difficult to value small increments of exercise, most, if not all, successful athletes work toward specific big goals. Today's short walk can be part of how you get ready to climb a mountain. If you want to race in a marathon-length triathlon, you have to do your homework. There's no skimping on training if that type of event is your goal.

Find a goal that really excites you. Then, enjoy the process of getting there. In setting goals that are attractive to you, you will help yourself to stay motivated. Do you want to be able to stay fit enough to climb your stairs easily during treatment? That can be a worthy goal. Do you want to stay strong enough so that you can carry your own groceries? Think for a minute about what might be some realistic goals for the next month or two. No goal is too humble if it is meaningful to you.

In the middle of treatment, it may sometimes be difficult to know what realistic goals might be. Perhaps you can talk with some cancer survivors in your community or online to see what others have experienced. You can review the profiles of cancer survivors in this book. Talk to a physical therapist, a sports trainer or a yoga teacher who has worked with cancer survivors. Whatever your goals might be, set them. It will give you something to aim for and a reason to keep that appointment to be active against cancer.

EQUATE EXERCISE WITH RELAXATION AND FUN

I almost never use the word "workout" in my conversations. I don't like it very much. First, it's vague. What activity is that: working out? I would rather run, ski, swim, or bike ride. Put a specific verb in the sentence and I'll get excited. Secondly, "working out" has the word "working" in it. That's not exactly a turn-on. Work? Being active in sports is supposed to be fun. Your activities provide a time for you to play. It's like recess for adults who like to be as happy as they can be.

One day when I was skiing, I was frustrated with my speed, and I was grumbling to myself about one thing or another. Then I heard some beginner skiers shouting "wa-hoo" during their inexpert attempts at skiing down a steep hill. I stopped and listened to their jubilation. I started laughing at myself! If having fun was the goal, those skiers with snow on their faces were winning. I, the ski racer, was losing. I re-set my goals immediately.

Having fun is a goal that I endorse. It's an attitude shift that I remind myself of routinely. I called ski racing my hobby to emphasize that it was for fun. Take your sport seriously, but just don't take it so seriously that you stop having fun!

Here's another tip: Don't use the word "hard" to describe a workout. I know a highly successful ski coach who has eliminated that word from his vocabulary and his team's. His team is disciplined, well trained, and motivated, but they don't label their activities or races as hard. Their superb race results come from commitment, effort, and practice, not from hard workouts because they don't do *any* of those. The racers don't associate difficulty with performing well. Good plan. By the way, "high intensity" is a good label for supposedly hard workouts.

You might think that you have to suffer to go fast. Not necessarily so. I will tell you a secret of aerobic athletes: Some of them are just as relaxed moving at top speed as you are moving more slowly. Some of them are even more relaxed than you are, actually. It's part of being efficient and effective.

EVALUATE YOUR OWN FATIGUE

Not all cancer survivors are alike in how much exercise they can do during their cancer treatment. You may begin your cancer journey already in fairly good shape or you may begin your cancer path less in-shape than you would like to be. You may have a more or less arduous course of treatment. Your ability to exercise may rise and fall during the ups and downs of your treatment and its side effects. All of these factors, and more, can affect your experience of fatigue.

In the course of five months, I had good days and bad; tired hours and less tired hours; days when I could go upstairs almost like normal; and days when I had to climb stairs slowly pausing at each new step for breath. Generally, however, I kept confident that I could do some exercise almost every day, whether I was tired or not.

My confidence came from my endurance sports background where I had learned that I could push myself even when I was tired. I was able to gauge how much exercise, during chemotherapy, felt like the right amount. I listened to my body. If I just felt slowed by lower blood counts, I exercised a small amount. I made sure not to push myself too hard or too long, but I was comfortable going for a short walk or a relaxing swim–even when

I was tired. I would just slow down the pace, rest if needed, and keep the distance short.

KEEP YOUR INTEREST UP

Let's look at a laundry list of suggestions for how to keep your interest level up. Exercise doesn't have to be the least bit dull. After you have achieved some fitness, you may want to branch out in any number of ways. Here are some options.

- Change your aerobic activity choice periodically.
- Learn new sports skills, games or activities.
- Change your exercise buddies or add some more.
- Mentor someone else in your chosen activity.
- Take a lesson in a sport you haven't tried before.
- Try outdoor sports.
- Take a class with other people.
- Enter a race or sign up for an athletic event.
- Go to new locations for your activities.
- Get passionate about one sport and learn to excel at it.
- Take dancing lessons.
- Try Wii-fit games or other similar games.
- Try racing or being part of a team.
- Exercise with children.
- Use a personal trainer to help expand your horizons.
- Get a new workout outfit, pair of shoes, or bike.
- Take an athletic vacation trip.
- Read inspiring sport biographies or sports magazines.
- Coach a sport.
- Volunteer at a race or a cancer fundraising sports event.

Whatever you do, find a way to make exercise enjoyable, day after day, month after month. Can I be blunt? If you get bored, it's up to you to fix it. Put some fun in your exercise and make it something you look forward to, please.

MORE FUN: BE ACTIVE TOGETHER

Just as I don't know any standout athletes who hate exercise, I also don't know any who only ever exercise alone. Most people who are routine exercisers share their exercise time with other people on occasions. There are running clubs, group hikes, cycling clubs, golf leagues, and all manner of team sports. Rare is the person who only ever works out alone. It simply is hard to stay motivated entirely alone one hundred percent of the time. Besides, it's fun to share a run, a bike ride, or a ski chairlift.

If you are feeling unwell during cancer treatment, it can be tempting to do your activity alone so that you can control your own pace. That strategy can work for some people. A solitary walking routine can be satisfying, but a walk with a friend can bring its own pleasures and rewards.

If you are currently going through cancer treatment, chances are pretty good that people ask you from time to time what they can do to help. They mean it: They want to help. You can say, "Would you go for a walk with me this Saturday morning? I don't walk very fast, but I would enjoy your company."

You might find someone from a cancer support group that you attend who wants to share a walk. Or you could do aerobic exercise with a group of other cancer survivors. You do this for free using DVDs for instruction, in a church basement or community space. You could help others by your example. That's a morale boost, for sure.

Although your loved ones, friends, or family may want to help you exercise during cancer recovery, you are ultimately the one who is charge of your exercise. Other people will let you down occasionally, despite good intentions. They'll be busy when they thought they had time. They will get a cold and stay away because of their germs. You want to count most on the only person you can control: yourself!

LET'S GO SHOPPING

People will exercise more often if they like their exercise outfits. Someone actually has studied that. You're welcome. Now you have a good reason to go shopping for workout clothes that you like. It's an investment in your good health and your cancer recovery. Can't afford much? Try a thrift store or bargain department store.

What makes a good exercise outfit? First, try to have wicking fabric on your shirts and, for women, in your sports bras. Fabrics can wick the sweat away from your body making you stay dry and smell sweeter. Plus, in cold temperatures, not having wet clothes clinging to you helps you avoid getting cold.

I would rank the overall fit and function of your outfit as very important. In biking, bike shorts have padding that helps protect you from saddle sores. If you don't like the look, ladies, buy a type with a skirt-like panel over the shorts. For running, you need comfort and lightweight clothes that don't restrict you. If you are new to buying sports clothing, go to a sports store, plead ignorance and ask for help.

The right clothes can help you tolerate any weather. Learn about rainwear, layers, Gore-Tex, Capilene, or whatever it takes to stay comfortable. And no, you don't ever need to wear Lycra tights if you don't want to.

Women can easily find a style sense that you enjoy. I thank goodness that I no longer have to wear dark blue wicking shirts only or buy a men's small to get the features that I want in outdoor gear. Try Title Nine Sports' store online or the womens' sporting clothes from Isis. Athleta, a women's sport and yoga clothing company, has excellent big and tall options. Capris or cute skirts with shorts built-in underneath (skorts) are popular active clothing options that flatter different shapes.

Do you want to announce that you're a cancer survivor? Try a Livestrong hat or t-shirt. You can channel the collective courage of the millions of cancer survivors in the world. Raymond, who was profiled here, called his Livestrong shirt his armor against cancer. I felt my yellow bracelet and Livestrong cap meant that I was a member in a big, brave, worldwide club of people who want to send cancer packing. Or you can wear the color that is associated with your type of cancer, if that sort of thing appeals to you. My color, teal, is often unfamiliar to people, but the popular colors are known.

OUTDOOR EXERCISE IS REVITALIZING

Get outside. Doing activities outdoors is rejuvenating and uplifting, and it is more so than time spent indoors at a gym or mall-walking. Again, a social scientist recently spent time to prove that obvious conclusion. I don't want to belabor the point. Most people, I think, already enjoy the outdoors. For me, being able to do outdoor sports accomplishes two things at once: I get all the benefits of the sports activities and I get to spend time in nature, out in the weather and sunshine. I love it! My life wouldn't have half of the joy that it does if I didn't step outdoors as often as I can.

If you are uncomfortable with outdoor exercise, look again at your reasons. Icy roads or dangerous areas can be problems. Perhaps you can think of some solutions. Perhaps you can walk with a dog, during different hours, with a friend, or use better shoes. You can add ice-gripping contraptions to your shoes, such as the brand called Yaktrax.

Consider trying something new outdoors. A kayaking adventure doesn't have to be difficult. Just paddle along in a two-person boat on a calm lake or river. Go with someone who knows how for the first few times. Or join a hiking group. You would be amazed how many hiking club members are just like you. Go birdwatching and then go for an extra walk in the woods. Maybe your outdoor exercise can begin in your yard or at the end of your driveway. Enjoy some fresh air and deep breathing.

CELEBRATE WITH EXERCISE

Who doesn't like a celebration? Use exercise as a part of how you celebrate completing milestones in your cancer recovery. Perhaps you will find a slow hike to a mountain summit to be your reward for making it through cancer treatment. One survivor interviewed for this book, Raymond, took a summertime trip to South America to catch up with some downhill skiing that he had missed during his winter of treatment. Others take celebratory runs or do races when they are feeling fit again.

When you are physically ready, set yourself up to do something special and memorable. Studies show that cancer survivors do well to set future goals. Why not make a great exercise goal a part of your plans? Be bold, get support and start planning.

CONSIDER RACING WHEN YOU ARE READY

If your health is good enough for you to do high intensity exercise or if you are willing to race at a slow pace, consider participating in a race. There are as many ways to look at racing, as there are contenders in a race. In truth, only a tiny percentage of people line up at the start with dreams of winning. Most people have their own agendas: do their best, have fun, keep a steady pace or finish faster than their ten-year-old does. You can even set several goals: one for your time, one that you are sure you can meet, and one just for fun.

Please understand that nearly all your competitors in a race are focused on doing their best, not on what you are doing. If you're not racing for the win, you shouldn't spend thirty seconds out of your race day thinking about what anyone else is doing or if they are judging you. They are probably not thinking about you at all, and if they are, well, they are probably thinking your t-shirt is a nice color or some other banal thought. Please, please, don't avoid racing. It can be a blast.

To build a great attitude about exercise, the best thing, in my opinion, is to do some competing. Having a race or other event on your calendar can be a great way to stay motivated with your usual exercise routine. To start racing, you sign up and then you show up. If you need to be convinced that you are welcome, go to a similar event first and volunteer to help. You will see people just like you competing and having fun! It's not a very well kept secret any more, but big races are very fun, social and wonderful for all levels of competitors.

Racing expertise and training plans, if you want them, can be found in magazines, clubs or from veteran racers. Most people will gladly give you advice from their own experience: as long as you ask after the race is over! Methodical, well-designed training plans help you to do your best.

Unfortunately, showing you how to build a great training plan is beyond the scope of this book, but you should know that adequate race preparation does not have to take any more time than the Sustaining Plan does. It depends on your event, your goal and your preferences, but you should be able to do a 5-km walk or run event based on your activity level from the Sustaining Plan. On a good day, jump in and try it.

Many cancer-related organizations have fundraising athletic events. There, if you are a cancer survivor, you are already a winner. These events tend to feel less competitive to beginning racers and very supportive, as well. Step into your new role and take it for a walk or a run. There is more information on these events in the last chapter.

ACTIVE SURVIVOR PROFILE: SHERRY

EXERCISE IS FUN AND POSSIBLY LIFE-SAVING

Sherry Daniels, a former high-ranking tennis player, ran Vermont's largest fitness center for almost twenty years. Staying fit has been a lifelong high priority for her. Her trim, energetic form at sixty-four years old makes her look like she has always been the picture of health.

"Exercise is fun," Sherry said during our interview. "It's what I do for a hobby."

Her activities include indoor morning workouts at home, where she does such things as stationary bike riding, Tae Bo, aerobic video workouts, or strength training with a Bow-Flex™. She gets at least 30 minutes of exercise every day and she does activities outdoors for longer periods of time on most weekends. Sherry was formerly "all about tennis," but in recent years, she finds that she likes more balance in her activities. She runs, rides her bike on country roads, cross-country skis, skates on her backyard ice at night, or puts on a headlamp to snowshoe after dark during winter.

Sherry's ability to use exercise as a positive outlet came in very handy when she faced her double cancer challenge. Sherry had not one, but two cancers, in quick sequence. She had just completed a lumpectomy for breast cancer, twelve weeks of chemotherapy and seven weeks of radiation, when she was diagnosed with stage III ovarian cancer. The ovarian cancer diagnosis led to major surgery and eighteen weeks of chemotherapy, during which she had an infusion every three weeks, repeated six times.

Many people would crumble mentally at such a double-load of cancer treatment: Sherry paced herself. She credits being in shape before cancer with helping her stay stronger throughout the multiple treatments and the overall ordeal.

During her treatment, although she didn't have the same energy level as normal, she had enough energy to do some exercise. The exercise, she believes, contributed positively to her coping ability and her recovery generally. Instead of running, she would walk, nearly daily. If she needed to, she took naps, then she would use the energy she did have to do some exercise.

Her doctors did not give her any specific exercise advice. She recalls them saying something like: "Don't overdo it." She did benefit from being part of a hospital-based twelve-week course on stress reduction. It taught her about relaxation techniques and included information on eating well, exercise, and coping with anxiety. Sherry felt that the course made a big difference in her ability to keep going.

"Of course you wonder if you're going to make it," Sherry admits.

Sherry had the usual reasons to wonder, plus one other poignant reason. She had lost her sister to a long cancer battle just years before her own cancers. After eleven years of being a cancer survivor with no further evidence of disease, Sherry wonders, today, if her fitness helped protect her from her genetic legacy until age fifty-two. It's a potent question because Sherry's younger sister, Ellie, was revealed to have advanced cancer at age forty-two.

"Was it my fitness that made a difference?" she wonders. "Did it offer me some kind of protection?"

No one can say for sure, but Sherry's devotion to fitness and exercise has never wavered—not before she had cancer twice and not since. Sherry is an accessible, encouraging role model for many women who are newly diagnosed with ovarian cancer. Long-time survivors of Stage III ovarian cancers are rare. In Sherry's small state of Vermont, if you have ovarian cancer, someone will probably mention her to you to give you hope. Her cancer history is publicly known. Sherry is active in the cancer community as an advocate and educator, and she is instrumental in support of the Eleanor B. Daniels Fund, a cancer support fund at a regional health care center. The fund helps educate ovarian cancer survivors, as well as promote advances in the treatment of the disease.

If you met Sherry, you would see the vibrant, caring, energetic person that she is. That she has taken care of her health, beaten cancer twice, stayed physically fit, and helped her community immensely is a tribute to her strength and to the legacy of love for her sister.

CHAPTER TEN

ADJUSTING YOUR ACTIVITIES DURING CANCER TREATMENT

What happens when you can't fulfill your original exercise plan? What if you are forced off schedule or have temporary limits due to health setbacks, medical treatment, or the side effects of treatment? You should adjust your activities accordingly. Although you need to be flexible in your exercise routine, you also want to continue to think of yourself as being on track with your exercise plan. Stick with your exercise agenda, even if you have certain limitations for a while.

The adjustments, discussed here, can help you continue being active, despite irregularities in your schedule. Rather than thinking of yourself as not exercising, you can frame your situation positively. After you make modifications to your original goals, you can be active in whatever ways are appropriate.

Remember, doing any exercise is meaningful to your health. Every little bit counts. If you can do some exercise, you will be that much closer to recovering your good health. Being active, even in small doses, will help your morale, as well. The advice to "avoid inactivity" should stay front and center during your cancer recovery, and let's admit it, forever.

THE ADJUSTMENTS

There are some simple ways to modify your activities: shorten, slow down, substitute, or skip. One adjustment is to shorten the length of time that you spend exercising. Secondly, you can make your pace of aerobic exercise slower. Your next option is to make substitutions. Do an alternative activity that better fits your condition that day or week.

If none of those adjustments seem possible, you can still honor your exercise time period by doing something symbolic that supports your healing. Perhaps listening to music and imagining yourself dancing would be uplifting, for example. Don't underestimate the power of visualizing movement. Last of all the adjustments, you can just skip exercising—and don't stress about it. Some days you need to just let it go. You'll know which days those are.

If you are in doubt about which activities to do, don't push yourself to do the most difficult of your options. Make a list of reasonable options, and then do the easiest, most appealing option. If you discourage yourself by pushing too hard, you are less likely to show up for your next exercise session. Discouraging yourself by making too big an effort is self-defeating.

Here are some detailed suggestions. Some of them are perfectly obvious, but a listing of the many options may help you see the range of choices. Remember, make a plan, and then adjust it as needed.

Shorten Your Aerobic Workout

Perhaps you have planned a 20-minute walk, but, today, you are feeling too poorly to do it. Can you do a 5-minute walk very slowly? Can you walk purposefully around your yard and see how you feel when you get started?

A slightly shorter walk than you might have planned can still be a constructive amount. Possibly, you can do two walks of half the usual length, if your stamina is the problem. You can walk more slowly than normal. You can rest for a few minutes part way along and then walk again.

The point is not to make yourself miserable but to see if you are able to do something active, rather than doing nothing at all. For some of you, it is easier to push yourself too hard and you may need to listen to your body and slow down or skip your walk. Others of you just need to encourage yourself to start walking and see how it goes.

Most people have some difficulty believing that a short walk of 5 or 10 minutes has any real merit. It does. It stimulates your immune system. Often, it can quell mild nausea. It can lift your mood. It can help your appetite. You may find you feel more energetic after exercise than you did before. Do a small amount of aerobic exercise, if you safely can, even if the efforts are slower and shorter than planned.

Slow Down

Sometimes all you need to do to adjust your plan is to slow down slightly during your aerobic workout. Listen to your body. If you have been walking at a certain pace, but today it is not comfortable, slow down. Push yourself to try a small dose of exercise if you feel up to it but don't push the pace to the maximum if you have any concerns.

There are many reasons that slowing down may be the right choice. Perhaps, if you are in active cancer treatment, you are experiencing the effects of having fewer red blood cells and less efficient oxygen-carrying capacity. It's perfectly fine to slow down and just do what feels good. For more information on coping with anemia and similar concerns, see chapter eleven.

If you are not familiar with exercising routinely, you may have a hard time knowing whether or not to push yourself and how much. Experienced athletes may find that they can judge how much to slow down; others of you may want to consult a personal trainer or physical therapist until you become more familiar with your body's signals during exercise.

If you are new to exercise, it can be hard to distinguish between signals to stop or signals that you should just slow down. Remember to check the list of contraindications to exercise in chapter five. You may even want to make a cheat sheet based on that list and keep it handy.

Substitute Swimming

If you have enough energy for something, but not much stamina, perhaps you can go for a swim and mostly float around. Swimming was my default activity for many days when my energy was low. I would float on my back and do a gentle elementary backstroke and glide along. This floating motion was so soothing.

You can do the breaststroke, sidestroke, or elementary bacstroke to relax and then to rest more, you can just float. Spending a short time swimming can rejuvenate you and provide enough aerobic activity for an immune-system boost. Best of all, you are bound to forget, briefly, that you are tired, feeling poorly, and discouraged. Swimming can be a wonderful tonic on a bad day.

Pedal a Stationary Bike

An exercise bike can be your best equipment choice if you need to easily control your exercise intensity. You can adjust your effort level easily, and you can stop any time you want to. On the other hand, you can do this aerobic exercise without going outdoors, if that helps. That feature can be appealing in winter. Instead of doing no exercise, try a short stationary bike ride. Even if you just pick up your heart rate briefly, it will be a victory.

Having a stationary bike in your home can be an ideal gift to yourself. With a home exercise bike, you can be active on whatever schedule suits you. You can do 15 minutes in the morning and 15 minutes in the evening. You can watch television while you ride it. For frugal people, exercise equipment such as stationary bikes become available on Craigslist frequently. Mine came to me for under one hundred dollars, that way. And, I must add, thank goodness for Netflix and Dick Van Dyke Show episodes. Mary Tyler Moore and Dick Van Dyke kept me smiling–and pedaling–through my knee rehab hours!

Do Strength Training and Stretching

If you want to do some exercise, but you can't do the scheduled aerobic activity, skip the aerobic menu for the day. Instead, try some gentle stretching, using yoga postures or stretches that you know. If the stretching goes well, maybe you can try some of your at-home weight-lifting program. Do as much or as little as you feel like. Sometimes if you don't feel like moving much, you can still enjoy some strength training.

Perhaps that amount of exercise will be enough to give you an uptick in wellness for the day. Rest a lot between efforts, if you need to. If you find you have more energy than you expected, do some dancing around the room or simply some arm movements in a flowing pattern while you remain seated. Enjoy the sensation of moving and using your body. No one is watching, so why not?

Do a Seated Workout

Ever heard of chair yoga? You can modify some yoga postures to do them in bed or in a chair. Or you can move your arms to music, raising your pulse somewhat. Experiment. See what is possible: leg raises, arm circles, lifting light weights, or some stretching. Any pleasant motion can be exercise that counts. Maybe you can sit on the edge of the bed and swing your legs. Sit-ups might work. Get creative and see what you can do.

A physical therapist may be able to advise you if you are going to be bed-ridden for a period of time. It's important to do what you can to maintain muscle tone, if at all possible.

Reduce the Intensity of Your Strength Workout

If you're going to skip your usual strength-training workout because of illness, injury, or fatigue, before you abandon it completely, consider modifying it. Is there something that you could tolerate doing in the strength-training category? Perhaps for one day, just doing your upper body or your lower body exercises would be sufficient. Perhaps you can do half the usual number of repetitions: instead of ten, try five of each movement. Perhaps you can just do push-ups but nothing more.

Delay Your Exercise Until You Feel Better

When I was recovering from surgery, a home nurse told me to keep in mind that a bad morning did not mean that I would have a bad day. I might have a good afternoon or a good evening. She suggested that feeling bad for an hour might not mean I would feel bad continuously all day. Healing is a process and it isn't the same all day, each day, nor is it always predictable. Her words stuck with me and I really took it to heart. If I had a morning exercise plan, but I couldn't do it, maybe I could make time in the evening. I tried to find the time of day when I felt the most motivated to exercise.

Sometimes when we're healthy, we know easily how to plan our days. When you have health troubles, you quickly learn to be flexible. Look for the times of day when your exercise plans might still work for you.

Skip Exercise for One Day or More

You will know when your treatment knocks you down so hard that you have to just rest up. Several of the people profiled in this book referred to taking a set number of days off after each chemotherapy infusion, for example. Try to retain your commitment to exercise by anticipating which day you can exercise again.

Perhaps you can use the time to write in a journal or call a friend who is supportive of your healing intentions. Nurture and care for yourself. Watch an uplifting movie about someone doing a sport that you admire or browse the Livestrong website for inspirational articles. Or watch a musical and imagine you are dancing. It really helps.

Try Eastern Traditions or Other Movement

Tai Chi, Chi Gong and related arts can be beneficial to your healing and alternatives to more vigorous exercise. If you want to do something very gentle, try these Eastern martial arts. Using a DVD for a guide, you can safely do them at home, if you're too tired to travel to a class. Alternatively, try free-style dancing to music that you find uplifting. Or while listening to music, sway and move your arms. You can move even if you are seated and in bed. Just enjoy it.

If you are low on energy, perhaps you can try to do some slow yoga, focusing on your breathing. Connecting to how you feel can feel good, even if you are feeling low. Try to connect with your intention to heal. See chapter twelve for more on these movement practices.

Use Gentle Yoga for Pain Relief and Relaxation

Consider doing some yoga poses that are completely relaxing. Fully being present in your body can be a gift, even if you are having some pain or difficulties. Sometimes being more present in your body allows the pain to be less bothersome than if you try to ignore your body. Relax with some yoga and try to find a peaceful moment amid the many moments of your day.

Symbolic Exercise: Try a Healing Visualization

If you are not able to do an aerobic activity, then a restful, relaxing harnessing of your mind's healing powers may be just what you need to stay encouraged. See chapter twelve for more ideas about healing meditation and related techniques. Healing visualizations can really help with pain, immune system function, and anxiety, among other things.

SET YOUR GOALS IN CONTEXT

To be dedicated to getting adequate exercise means thinking about your exercise plans day by day. It also means thinking about your exercise plans for a week at a time, a month at a time, and a year at time. If you are in active cancer treatment and using exercise to help your body fight cancer, then you are probably not going to be at your fittest. Accept that and keep it in context. Your goal is to get healthy again and maybe in one year's time to be at the level of fitness that you crave.

Sometimes, for an entire period of treatment, which can be many months long, you will be active with a goal of not losing too much strength and fitness. Instead of seeing that situation as non-optimal, see yourself as nurturing your return to health. Go easy on your regrets and on yourself. Most cancer patients who are in treatment slow down. They modify activities; they hang on. When that is the best that you can do, it's meaningful!

WHERE TO GET PERSONALIZED HELP

You may want to solicit personalized information on some details of your exercise plans from an expert whom you can meet with. You may do best if that person can talk with your doctor, as well. The ACSM or your treating physician may be able to help you find a knowledgeable physical therapist or personal trainer in your area. Ask for help from your cancer center or hospital. The new specialty of oncology rehab is growing. You can also ask a home health agency or a fitness center what they know about oncology rehab specialists in your area. The Livestrong Foundation sponsors exercise programs at many community YMCAs. There is more information about their programs in chapter thirteen.

WORK WITH YOUR TREATMENT SCHEDULE

Many cancer treatment protocols eventually reveal themselves to be nearly predictable, so you may find that you can plan ahead. You can skip certain activities on certain days and then go back to your original exercise plan.

Your nurses or doctors may also be able to give you some guidance based on their experiences with other patients. Likewise, you may find a personal trainer, physical therapist, or even a community member who can help you plan around your treatment schedule. Sometimes just knowing that you will feel more like exercising by next Tuesday is enough to keep you on track and motivated.

FATIGUE, ACTIVITIES, AND YOUR AGENDA

You may want to consider this question: Are your job duties or usual daily activities a source of overall exhaustion to you? Are you trying to do everything that you did before cancer during your recovery or treatment period? If you find that your schedule is overwhelming and that exercise is the first thing that you skip, consider making adjustments to your responsibilities. Make your cancer recovery your top priority while you are in treatment, if that is feasible. Do give the issue of your priorities some thought.

In one of the survivor profiles, Denise mentioned that during her second episode of breast cancer, she stopped working at her job in order to focus on her healing. Another person, Sherry, mentioned a similar plan after her second different kind of cancer. Could it be that if you have already experienced the rigors of treatment once, you can better judge just how much time to devote to healing and self-care? Think about it.

STAY FOCUSED ON BEING ACTIVE

Attitude counts for a lot. Are you unable to exercise or just unable to be very active today? Are you adjusting your exercise plan or giving up? Are you looking forward to getting back to exercising or are you just relieved to have an excuse for skipping your walk today?

Try to be positive in your approach to exercise. If the beginning of the week is bad, maybe the end of the week will be good. If the morning is bad, maybe the afternoon will be good. With any luck, you will be able to enjoy your activities often enough for frequent rewards.

ACTIVITY PLANNING WORKSHEET

Are you running into problems doing what you need to do for exercise? This set of questions is designed the help you problem-solve. Take a look at the questions and if you need to address any concerns, ask a friend or other person to help you do further problem-solving. Knowing what is holding you back is the first step toward fixing it.

1. What are my favorite ways to be active, move, and enjoy exercise?

2. What appeals to me right now for activities, given my limitations?

3. Are there special adjustments that I can make to help me stay active?

4. What other new or different activities am I willing to try?

5. What time of day is best for me to fit in my activities?

6. If I'm still getting treatment, what is my schedule and how can I plan activities around it?

7. What comes up when I wonder if I will actually exercise as planned?

8. What can I do to succeed in the face of those obstacles?

9. Who will be supportive of my exercise activities? Include new and familiar people, clubs, supporters, and people at your fitness center, if any.

10 What special medical concerns do I have?

11. Who will help me with my medical concerns and when will they help?

12. What is my one-month goal for exercise? Three months? Six months?

13. The best way that I can stay motivated to exercise is...

14. My slogan for being active against cancer is...

15. How can I be part of the cancer survivor community to get support for exercise?

※ ※ ※

ACTIVE SURVIVOR PROFILE: BETSY

STAYING ON THE TEAM

Like many serious, successful high school athletes, Betsy hoped to use her proficiency at three high school sports to be recruited to a college athletic program. She excelled in hockey, lacrosse, and field hockey. Betsy faced an unusual obstacle, however: she spent most of her critical junior year on the bench, not from an injury, but as the result of going through seven months of arduous chemotherapy for Stage IV Hodgkin's lymphoma. Despite this hurdle, Betsy was recruited to play sports at the University of Vermont (UVM). She has been cancer free for six years. Here is her story.

Betsy's UVM field hockey coach, Nicki, had seen Betsy's hockey skills and talent during Betsy's healthy sophomore year of high school. Nicki had kept in touch with the young standout athlete. As Nicki would later recall, Betsy was having a lot of pain in her legs during her junior year in high school. The doctors could not figure out what was going on. They changed her shoes. Then they gave her orthotics, thinking this would solve the leg pain. Finally, Betsy was diagnosed with Hodgkin's disease. She would need a long course of treatment and she would need to beat the odds.

Betsy says that she coped with her cancer challenge by trying to hold onto her normal life as much as possible. However, "normal" for Betsy meant playing three sports, and her fatigue—and later her blood counts—would not allow her to continue as a full-time player. Despite having been in the top group in ice hockey, Betsy, during treatment, could only run drills in practice sessions. She could not skate in any contact drills, that is, those drills that allowed hitting. Additionally, she had to pace her efforts to match her fatigue levels.

Rest doesn't relieve fatigue from chemotherapy because the fatigue is based more on low blood counts (both red and white blood cells) than on inadequate sleep or muscle fatigue from exercise. Betsy was tired walking up a set of stairs, something that she had never experienced before. Even though she started to have clear scans (that is, no cancer in evidence) halfway through her treatment, Betsy was increasingly fatigued from the chemotherapy. She couldn't always skate.

Eventually, her high school coaches made her an assistant coach. This role gave Betsy a new reason to be at practice. She was included in coach's meetings. She needed to study the game while it was played by her teammates so that she could contribute her observations. An upside to her coaching role was that she learned to "see the game" better and understand it more as she had more time to observe strategy.

It would take Betsy almost a full year after the end of treatment to get back to her normal energy levels; by this time, she was a senior in high school. Nicki recruited Betsy, who went on to play field hockey at UVM, where Betsy was a major contributor to the success of her team.

After her outstanding college sports ended, Betsy took up running. With characteristic determination, she soon was training for marathon races. She joined the Team in Training (TNT), a training program in support of survivors of blood cancers. Ever modest, she told no one whom she trained with about her cancer history until after she completed her first marathon with TNT.

Betsy is now using her passion for health care in her studies for a master's degree in nursing from Columbia University. She wants to be able to help others when they face their cancer challenges. She will be a remarkable help to cancer patients, just as she was a great team player. Having been a positive force in her own healing, Betsy is a bright spirit who did, indeed, beat the odds.

CHAPTER ELEVEN

SPECIAL MEDICAL CONCERNS DURING CANCER TREATMENT

This chapter presents information about fairly common concerns that you might have during treatment and cancer recovery. These medical concerns may influence the type or amount of exercise that you do. Not all cancer survivors will need all of this information, so read about the topics that interest you. After reading about these issues, you should discuss any of your concerns with your treating professionals. Remember to be a proactive patient. Discuss your medical concerns with your doctor or medical treatment team before you begin exercising and discuss them again as your condition changes.

BLOOD COMPOSITION CONCERNS

If you are in active treatment for cancer, it is routine for your medical team to monitor your blood counts, as they are called. They will advise you of any medical concerns that result from your changes in blood components. Chemotherapy and radiation can alter your blood composition, as can cancer itself. Sometimes these changes are cyclical. Your blood counts may trend towards normal before the next treatment, but it is also common for your counts to change over the course of months if you have a long treatment protocol. The blood composition may improve slightly but not come back to normal near the end of months of treatment, for example.

When your medical team reviews your routine blood counts, they evaluate three types of blood counts (among other things): your red blood cell count; your white blood cell count; and your platelet count. Please ask your physician for more information about your blood counts because the following information is general in nature. Your physician will analyze your blood count information in the context of your overall health status, treatment plans and prognosis. That kind of analysis is, of course, beyond the scope of this book's presentation. Here are some basic facts about blood count numbers.

Anemia

Anemia is a condition where your blood has too few red blood cells, not the optimal number. A red blood cell carries hemoglobin, and hemoglobin is the chemical that oxygen attaches to. Oxygen circulates in your blood so that it can reach your muscles and allow them to function. If you have anemia, and thus, have too few red blood cells, you have too few molecules of hemoglobin, and less than the optimal amount of oxygen circulating to reach your muscles.

Your lowered oxygen-carrying capacity of your blood can make you feel out of breath because of the lowered volume of oxygen in your blood. For example, an activity, such as climbing a flight a stairs, may become something that you must do slowly, when you used to do it easily. You may need to breathe in deliberately, resting on each step up, as your body tries to get adequate oxygen to your muscles.

The American Cancer Society guidelines suggest that you do not exercise if you have anemia. Other medical professionals, including Charlene Gates, R.N., of the Dartmouth-Hitchcock Medical Center's Norris Cotton Cancer Center (NCCC), have suggested a different approach. In NCCC's video for breast cancer survivors, the presenters state: Slow down if your hemoglobin level is below 8.0. This score means you are anemic, but you may be able to do exercise such as walking, if you slow your pace adequately. You should ask your own treating medical professionals to help you interpret your number relative to any risks to you might have with exercise. (There are many numbers below 8.0, I realize, and the advice here does not pertain to severe anemia at significantly lower numbers.)

If you have mild anemia, except for your experience of fatigue, there is not a specific or severe health risk to doing some aerobic activity within your comfort range. For example, you might naturally slow down your pace walking up the stairs, but you can still walk up the stairs. You could also, in the same fashion, go for a walk, albeit slowly, and stop to rest when you needed to.

If you are able to do some very low intensity exercise, you can maintain some level of aerobic fitness and conditioning. As a result, your episodes of low red blood cell counts may feel more easy to bear and more tolerable. Because activity has so many benefits, it is important to not avoid activity too often. Be aware that you do not need to rest completely, for example, if you have a slightly lowered red blood cell count.

Another possible benefit of continuing to do some light, appropriate activities when you have slightly lowered red blood cell counts is that your body, in response to your activity, may be stimulated to increase red blood cell production. This is an area of speculation and current research, but it seems, on the surface, to make sense. When visiting geographic areas of high altitude, the body quickly adapts to the reduced oxygen in the air by making more red blood cells, for example.

Speaking of high altitude, let's consider athletes who exercise without optimal oxygen levels in their blood. When high altitude mountaineers climb Mount Everest, they have less oxygen available to them in the thin mountain air of 30,000 feet. Consider what high-altitude climbers do to cope with thin air–besides carrying supplemental oxygen. They slow down. They take a step; rest; then take another. It looks like slow motion. If you walk up a flight of stairs slowly because of your low red blood cells, you may feel tired, but you aren't likely to do harm to yourself. You can do it.

Here is another example. Many runners challenge their bodies to move fast, demanding more oxygen to reach their muscles quickly. If they run faster than their fitness has prepared them for, they can start to struggle with being out of breath, and they have to slow down. Runners, from casual ones to professionals, do that frequently without worrying about causing any significant damage. It's not much different than having a slightly low red blood cell count.

Naturally, no one wants you to climb in the Himalayas during cancer treatment. Here's my personal experience. I did hike up a 4,000-foot-plus mountain several months into my five-month chemotherapy course. Other days, I was just as happy walking on a flat dirt road. In either case, I rested frequently, sitting down. My point is that you may not have to stop all exercise the moment your red blood cell count is less than optimal. If you give up on mild or moderate aerobic exercise too easily, you can hurt your fitness, your red blood cell production, and your overall cancer recovery.

When discussing red blood cell counts, your doctor may suggest a prescription medicine to increase your red blood cell production. Please do some good research if you are being offered such medication. Perhaps you can get a medical second opinion so that you have adequate information about some of the complexities involved with these medications. They are not without serious possible side effects and possible long-term risks. The most serious concern is that the medications may stimulate tumor growth. The medications can be life-saving and crucial to your recovery, but sometimes they are offered when their use is not strictly necessary. When you seek more information, pay attention to the source of that information. You will have to make up your mind.

My own personal decision was to avoid this class of medications. I tried to stimulate the healing processes of my body with exercise, nutrition, rest, and other types of self-care during chemotherapy. I preferred a certain amount of fatigue from mild anemia rather than to use medication that I was not comfortable with. I had mild anemia from which I rebounded quickly. Your situation may be different. This class of medication is in wide use and has real benefits when it is needed. (By the way, perhaps you have heard of athletes abusing EPO for advantage. That drug is in the same class discussed here.)

Neutropenia

If you are neutropenic, you have a lowered count of the type of white blood cells known as neutrophils. This condition affects your immune system function. If you are neutropenic or otherwise have compromised immune function, you are at increased risk of getting an infection, and your body's immune system may not handle the infection as well as it normally would. Severe infections become more likely, possibly including life-threatening infections that require hospitalization and treatment.

Although neutropenia can result in severe illness, there is a range of numbers reflecting your neutrophil count. The numbers range from optimal through slightly lowered down to quite dangerously low. The risk of health problems increases the farther the numbers are from normal. Ask your doctor to put your numbers in context for you.

For example, do many patients who have numbers like yours fare well and see their numbers easily rebound? Or is your number indicating a very serious risk? Become familiar with the range of numbers, rather than just thinking that anything lower than ideal is automatically very dangerous.

When your medical team advises you to stay away from crowds in public and limit your risk of infection because you are neutropenic, they are trying to protect your health. You may want to avoid going to work out at a gym because of exposure to other people's germs. On the other hand, perhaps you are still going shopping at the grocery store, and you are in contact with children, friends, and family, despite neutropenia. Perhaps going to the gym could be as safe as going to the grocery store—or safer. Try to go to the gym when it is not crowded. Wipe clean all surfaces with disinfectant before your use. You can limit your direct contact with people while there. If you make those accommodations, perhaps going to the gym is worth the limited risk.

Only your doctor knows your complete health profile, but you can ask which specific conditions are of concern for you and why. If you are given a broad statement such as "stay out of crowded places like the gym," try to ask more questions.

A short outdoor stroll away from other people may be the best answer if your risk of infection is high. Perhaps you can use home exercise equipment instead of going to a gym. Ask your doctor what solutions have worked for other patients like you.

Your medical team knows about a type of medication that can reduce your risk of becoming neutropenic, or treat you if you are already neutropenic. These drugs, although improved upon compared to a decade ago, are notorious for causing bone pain in many patients. They are also somewhat controversial because of fears of long-term negative effects. You will want to make a well-considered decision about using them. Ask questions. Do some extra reading about the drugs' side effects, their mechanisms, and their risks. Treating neutropenia with medications can be life-saving. Prophylactic use of this type of medication can prevent neutropenic fevers and, in large studies, its use shows a reduction in mortality from neutropenia. However, a subset of patients may be able to refrain from using this type of medication if their white blood cell counts are adequate.

Additionally, please note that your white blood cell counts are not the only indicators of reduced immune system function. Your resistance to infection depends on multiple factors, including your immunoglobulin levels. For example, patients who have had bone marrow transplants or stem cell transplants may have weakened immunity, despite normal blood counts. As always, ask your doctor for more information about how you should interpret your blood counts.

Low Platelet Count

Follow your doctor's advice about exercising when you have a low platelet count. Concerns and issues are similar to those of low white or red blood cells, but a low platelet count can lead to problems with blood coagulation (similar to clotting).

FATIGUE AND EXHAUSTION

If you miss some sleep and are tired the next day, you can usually recover your sense of energy by catching up on your sleep. Doing a small amount of exercise in normal health when sleepy won't harm you. If you are doing a long, high-intensity event, your performance will suffer. For example, a well-rested marathon runner, all things being equal, will be faster than a poorly rested one. The day after a big race, most athletes will be tired from the effort. They use the next days, weeks, or months to recover from that kind of fatigue.

Cancer patients play a whole different game when it comes to fatigue. It's much more complicated. First, fatigue during treatment has various sources, which can include: low red blood cell counts from side effects of drugs; low white blood cell counts from side effects; and digestive disturbances like vomiting leading to poor or no food intake. You can also be fatigued from the stress of the chemotherapy and its cumulative toll on your body's functioning. You can have fatigue from the burden of having cancer cells in your body. You can be fatigued from insomnia that was caused by anxiety or drug side effects. These sources of fatigue can mix and mingle so that you are tired for a variety of reasons.

With all these sources of fatigue, how do you know when to push yourself off the couch or out of bed to do even a short walk?

When is it okay to exercise if you are tired? When is it good for you or bad for you? First, go back to the initial list of precautions in chapter five. If any apply, do not exercise. Second, if you feel that exercise would be so dangerous that you are scared something bad would happen, do not exercise.

You can ask your doctor to assign you to physical therapy if you need assistance. Maybe you would feel safe if you had a structured, supervised program to get you started with a modest program like walking on a treadmill. Perhaps you need to begin that way in order to get comfortable.

In most cases, you can do a small amount of exercise safely if your fatigue is from slightly lowered blood counts or from mild gastro-intestinal upsets that don't make you dehydrated, woozy, or weak. Try a short duration of exercise such as 5 minutes, and only increase your exercise period by 5 minutes each day.

Do not attempt to exercise to the level of exhaustion during cancer treatment. Exercising moderately on a regular schedule is easier for your body to handle. You need to nurture your own healing, not exhaust yourself. Consider exercise as beneficial as long as your fatigue does not worsen from your activities.

During relatively long courses of chemotherapy, many patients feel fatigued constantly as they reach the middle or end of their treatment period. Although it is discouraging to feel this way, you may be someone who can still safely exercise. If you have no other contraindications to exercise, you may find that doing 30 minutes of easy aerobic activity makes you feel better, despite some ongoing fatigue.

If you feel tired, a small amount of light-intensity exercise may renew your energy levels. Exercise can provide short-term immediate relief from fatigue and that relief can be your daily incentive to exercise. The fatigue from chemotherapy or radiation may return the same day, but you could have pleasant interval where you feel good. If you can associate your exercise with feeling good, you will be more likely to stick with exercise and reap its other many anti-cancer benefits.

One important study showed that fatigue levels, after completing chemotherapy for breast cancer, were less for those who had exercised during treatment. Exercise also benefited patients' health after treatment ended. Fatigue was less, one year later, for the group who exercised during treatment compared to a sedentary group. Why this happens is not completely medically understood yet. It's okay not to wait until they figure it out, I think.

LYMPHEDEMA

Lymphedema is the swelling of tissue caused by changes in the function of your lymph system. As a typical example, a breast cancer patient who had many lymph nodes in her armpit removed may have chronic swelling from a lack of return of lymph fluid back up from her arm. The swelling itself is uncomfortable, ranging from bothersome to very painful, and it can have further negative effects on function.

For many years, the conventional medical wisdom was to discourage patients with lymphedema from weight lifting or other strenuous exercise that involved the affected limbs or area of the body with lymphedema. The concern was that vigorous exercise of a body part affected by lymphedema would have negative effects. That outdated concern has been replaced by better understanding of exercise and lymphedema.

The current medical thinking is simply that exercise can help lymphedema. It can help to prevent it and it can help to moderate it. In presenting to a seminar at the 2010 Breast Cancer Conference in Stowe, Vermont, Charlene Gates discussed a comprehensive study from 2010, of a type called a Cochrane's review. This medical report included a review of all studies on the subject of lymphedema and cancer recovery. Her summation was: "There is no evidence that exercise results in patients' developing arm lymphedema."

Exercise, in the right amounts and of the right difficulty, can very likely help you with lymphedema if you are afflicted with it. As Ms. Gates explained in the seminar, after lymphedema has become stable, a slowly progressive program of exercise, including weight lifting, has good benefit. Seek personalized professional advice from trained professionals on how to work with lymphedema. They can help you with issues such as: use of compression stockings or garments; how much exercise to do; how often; and what type.

NAUSEA

If you are battling severe nausea that is keeping you from exercise that you might otherwise be able to do, ask your doctor if there are more effective medications that might control your nausea better. Ask for a consult with another doctor to pursue this question, if necessary. There are a variety of drugs available. Work with your team so that you find something effective.

There are also a number of very safe and reasonable home remedies available, such as trying to keep eating small amounts rather than waiting only for meal-time to eat. You can also suck on peppermint, ginger, or plum candies when queasy, and you can take soothing teas with peppermint or ginger. Investigate to find remedies that might work for you. There is a lot of information available on this important topic.

Exercise in the short-term may quell mild nausea. For example, if you feel just slightly nauseated and do not want to eat for fear of throwing up, try a short walk of 5 minutes at a gentle pace or going up and down stairs a few times. This brief activity may be enough to quell your nausea so that you can eat a small amount, and then the food may help further reduce your nausea so that you are more comfortable. Activity can help the nausea not arrive, not be as severe, go away altogether, or not be as bothersome.

If your throwing up is imminent or your nausea is very severe by some other measure, you should not exercise. Again, be reasonable and don't exercise if you are at risk of hurting yourself.

OSTEOPOROSIS

Osteoporosis involves the weakening of bones due to mineral deficiencies. The extent of osteoporosis can vary and can be measured by a bone density scan. Mild osteoporosis or osteopenia, which is a deficiency that is milder than osteoporosis, can often benefit from weight-bearing activity or appropriate level of strength training. However, if you have moderate to severe osteoporosis, you may be at a risk for fractures.

You may have increased osteoporosis risk as the result of surgical menopause, from medically induced menopause, or from chemotherapy's lowering of your estrogen levels. Osteoporosis can also come from radiation treatment in some cases, or from hormone-blocking regimens, which are used for some breast cancers, some prostate cancers, or other cancers. The ACSM's *Exercise Guidelines for Cancer Survivors* notes that "multiple myeloma patients should be treated as if they have osteoporosis."

Discuss your health status in this regard with your doctor. Your family doctor may also be a source of information on dealing with osteoporosis risk.

PERIPHERAL NEUROPATHY

Some patients who receive chemotherapy with certain drugs are prone to developing peripheral neuropathy. Peripheral neuropathy means nerve damage in the hands or the feet, those being at the periphery of your body. Sensation in our bodies relies on nerves, both large and small. The small nerves farthest from our core, those nerves in our hands and feet in other words, are sometimes injured by chemotherapy agents.

Neuropathies can be mild or severe, short-lasting, or permanent. They can involve pain, numbness, funny sensations or a combination of these. You may experience a slight bit of numbness in your fingertips or tingling sensations in your fingers and on the soles of your feet. More severely, you might experience noticeable pain or total numbness your hands and feet. In worse cases, you can have trouble using your fingers for lack of sensation and trouble with walking because of balance problems originating with your numbed feet.

In some patients, peripheral neuropathy that develops, for example, late in treatment, will go away gradually over the next few months or up to about a year after treatment ends. Other times the peripheral neuropathy can be permanent, require changes in lifestyle, and be debilitating.

Ask your doctor what you can expect. The type of chemotherapy that you receive influences the results and your doctor will be familiar with your general risk. Unfortunately, your doctor is not likely to know exactly what you may experience because patient experiences vary. You will likely hear statistics about different outcomes, and you will need to wait and see how your symptoms progress or resolve.

If you are active with a walking program and have significant nerve problems in your feet, you need to evaluate whether or not you are at risk of falling. You should ask for some input from your medical team about your relative risks. If falling is a significant risk, then you should choose other activities like using an elliptical trainer or an exercise bike. However, a very mild amount of peripheral neuropathy may be tolerated during exercise.

Peripheral neuropathy changes can sometimes be treated with medication to reduce pain. Currently, no medications are available that treat the causes of peripheral neuropathy, but trials are underway on new drugs. You might also look into some over-the-counter supplements that are unproven but perhaps non-damaging and potentially helpful.

To help you evaluate the extent of your problems, you can get a consult with a neurologist for special testing of your nerves and an evaluation of the extent of your problem. Unfortunately, for some people who need a long course of chemotherapy with certain agents or a second round of chemotherapy for a recurrence of their disease, peripheral neuropathy damage can become severe and limit treatment options. It can worsen to the degree that the chemotherapy must be changed to avoid the offending agents.

Keep an eye out for information on any new supplements or medications to treat peripheral neuropathy. Research is pending on how to keep good nerve function, a goal of diabetics as well as chemotherapy patients.

❋ ❋ ❋

ACTIVE SURVIVOR PROFILE: STEPHANIE

RESTORING HER HEALTH AND RACING FOR A CAUSE

Stephanie Fraser, forty-eight years old, likes to combine her athletic events with a fundraising goal. She calls it having "dual goals," and the extra impetus of raising money for a good cause makes the training and racing more meaningful. She not only sets a goal for the speed of her race, but she also sets a fundraising goal. When she rode her bicycle one hundred miles, for a Livestrong Challenge event, her goals were a finish time of eight hours and fundraising an amount of five thousand dollars. She met both goals. Dramatically, her race was six months after completing arduous chemotherapy for ovarian cancer.

Stephanie was "over the cancer" after that race, she said in a recent interview. She's not being flip. In her day job, Stephanie is a social worker who helps patients who have cancer receive necessary financial and other support. She's respectful of cancer, but Stephanie is also a long-time survivor of kidney disease. She had her first kidney transplant in high school. After completing her cancer treatment, Stephanie knew that she was going to need a second kidney transplant. Staying well until she could get one was going to be a fight, and it was going to be her main focus for the foreseeable future. Stephanie had to be cancer-free for three years before she would be eligible.

Stephanie says that exercise was her way to cope when she was in cancer treatment. She walked an average of two hours every

139

day. After treatment ended, she rode her bike in preparation for the century ride. When she was waiting for a kidney transplant, her routine exercise helped her feel a sense of control over her health. She says that if she had stopped exercising, she felt that she would have gone downhill.

In fact, exercise has helped Stephanie all her life. As a young kidney transplant survivor, she participated in national and international Transplant Games as a cyclist, earning victories many times. For over two decades, she continued to participate in cycling races at the Transplant Games with impressive results.

After three cancer-free years, Stephanie had her second kidney transplant in 2008. The donated kidney came from a colleague, to whom she remains very grateful. Stephanie did her second Livestrong ride six weeks after she was allowed back on her bike after her kidney transplant. Currently, she "wants to shift gears and focus more on living organ donation where there has been a shortage of living donors." She wants to help more kidney donors be able to afford the cost of making a kidney donation. "No one has ever done that before," she says. To other people, that task might intimidate others, but Stephanie has been doing singular, impressive things most of her life.

Stephanie tells her story at cancer conferences and workshops: "I try to give people hope," she says. By example, she certainly does.

CHAPTER TWELVE

LET YOUR MIND HELP YOU HEAL

D o you find cancer's impact on your life stressful? Yes, that is a rhetorical question. Fortunately, you can benefit from using mind-body techniques and reduce some of your stress proactively. Relieving stress is a great way to advance recovery, a fact that many doctors are aware of now. The mind and the body are not separate. You can evoke healing with the mind's powers, using many mind-body techniques. This chapter will introduce you to some well-known stress reduction techniques such as guided visualizations, affirmations, yoga, and breathing exercises. If exercise is your main stress reliever, you can use these mind-body options on days when you cannot exercise.

Please keep an open mind. Trust your own experience more than your first reaction to a written description of a new technique. Many things that sound silly at first can actually be helpful when you try them. It's possible to benefit from using these techniques the very first time that you try them.

In this chapter, I also include some thoughts about keeping a good attitude toward healing and exercise. Coping skills are obviously very personal, but I have included some things that helped me. Perhaps some of my observations will resonate with you.

BE CAREFUL WITH LABELS

While I was going through cancer treatment, I was careful not to call myself "sick." I didn't feel tip-top and I suffered from many side effects, but I chose not to label myself as sick. I said, "I'm facing a cancer challenge right now." "I have some limits due to my cancer treatment." "I'm recovering from cancer." Or "I don't feel one hundred percent well because of some effects of my chemo."

With those words, I always left room for myself to be "not sick." I always left room for the side effects to wax and wane. I always left room for my recovery of my health. I never "wrote off" the whole summer. I had good days, good hours, good moments, and good times. I did not cast myself as merely sick and that decision, I think, helped me to be able to exercise and enjoy myself on many occasions.

FIND A SLOGAN

All the devoted recreational athletes whom I have met love to exercise. Time doing sports serves as a refuge from petty daily stresses and concerns.

I see my time exercising as time of renewal, time for relaxing, and time for serenity. I have used daily runs as tonics for depression, cures for a broken heart, and escapes from stress. I have run to feel free, jubilant, and natural. When doing my sports activities, I can relax and be free from negative thoughts. When I'm in motion, I often feel powerful, wonderful, and alive. I see my exercise time as a time when I get to be completely happy. For a while, I called the time that I spent running "my hour of joy."

What meaning can you give exercise? I almost titled this book "Exercise Beats Cancer." It sounded so empowering to me. If you want to think of your exercise time like that, please do! No one can argue with you. "Live strong" is a pretty good slogan, too. Is it taken? I'm just suggesting that you look for the meaning that you want to give to your exercise. Find out what works for you.

CHOOSING POSITIVE SELF-TALK

When I wanted to get back in shape, many years ago, so that I could do some ski racing, I started by running every day. Because I was less fit than I liked to be, I would think of discouraging things in my mind. One day, spontaneously, I stopped right in my tracks when I heard myself thinking: "I'm no good at this." I just stopped and stood still. I knew I had to change my thinking. Life was hard enough. Why beat up on myself during my exercise time?

Right then and there, I decided that I would only say nice things in my head while I was running. I remember the exact spot where I stood; it was a life-changing moment for me. I literally trained myself to disallow negative thoughts when I was running, by stopping if I became negative. I reinforced the positive thoughts and repeated certain positive phrases as I ran.

Guess what? I love exercise and I'm very happy when I'm doing it. I say all sorts of nice things to myself when I'm working out or racing. Actually, in races, I'm even more positive. I don't have time for a negative thought during a race; it would take seconds or minutes off my time. Coaches call this phenomenon "positive self-talk."

In my mind, practicing positive self-talk is also a great way to enjoy your whole life more. The habits of positive self-talk can also help you get through your cancer recovery. If you have ever derided positive thinking, your cancer challenge might be your opportunity to give it a re-think. During your exercise time, you can practice being kind and encouraging to yourself. You get immediate feedback. If you think, "This is hard" then the effort feels onerous. If you think, "This is fun," then you are well on your way to having fun.

As a result of racing and training with positive self-talk, I was already good at positive thinking when I received my cancer diagnosis. I didn't deny that I was scared, but I tried to keep my spirits up by thinking that I could recover my health. When I focused on a long-term good outcome, it was a lot easier to handle the daily trials. Please try positive self-talk.

SET YOUR GOALS HIGH

It's true in sports that you generally need to set a high goal in order to achieve it. People rarely take first place if they have only planned to finish in the middle of the pack. You usually have to imagine that you can win in order to put forth the effort it takes to train well and actually win.

Is this true for cancer recovery generally? I don't know for sure, but setting a high goal, like a full recovery, is mentally helpful. Why not try for a great recovery? It may help you handle the ups and downs better if you look towards your goal. Today might be a miserable day along the path towards a complete recovery. Even people with so-called bad odds do make recoveries. Count yourself among the ones who might be fortunate, as long as you can. You don't need to be a Pollyanna type to believe that you want to recover from cancer.

HEALING IMAGERY

One day when I had recovered enough from my abdominal cancer surgery, I went out on my local road and began running. I'm a lifelong runner, so it was a nice reunion between the lifting of my feet and the happiness in my heart. I had recently received my first dose of chemotherapy and the strangeness of the chemical infusion was on my mind. I was scared about cancer, for sure. Very scared.

Spontaneously, I came up with a jingle. I fit the rhythm of the words to the striking of my feet on the ground and added a faint melody. *"All the cells with bad instructions go away. All the cells with good instructions shout hooray!"*

These few words became my jingle to use throughout five months of chemotherapy. The words were my mantra, if you will. I pictured cancer cells as cells with bad instructions. They were trying to reproduce without having good functional roles like healthy cells do. I pictured the chemotherapy making the cancer cells go away and I imagined the good cells were happy and celebrating.

Call it a jingle, a mantra, or a positive healing image. Whatever you call it, it's great to have a positive image for a scary treatment like chemotherapy. It's even better, I think, if you can make the image rhyme and set it to the rhythm of your favorite exercise like walking or running. You may borrow my jingle, if you don't have one of your own.

You can also use positive imagery, mantras, or affirmations while you are not exercising, such as when you are receiving an infusion, struggling with pain, or lying sleepless with side effects some night. You might want to look into more formal mantra use or chanting to go with your yoga practice.

One book that I like is *Guided Imagery for Self-Healing* by Martin Rossman, M.D. In the resources section, I also list his audio recordings of guided visualizations, which I have found very helpful.

BE OPEN TO AFFIRMATIONS

Some people run scared from affirmations because they think that affirmations are merely wishful thinking. They don't have to be. Affirmations can describe actual possibilities for positive outcomes. I don't like to say anything that I don't believe, so I make my affirmations very carefully. You can be accurate and affirming at the same time. With some practice, it's easy to do.

Start with one of your worst fears or most negative thoughts. Write down one thing that you are struggling with. Then, find a way to reframe the exact same concern in a positive manner that you can believe in. For example, "I'm afraid chemotherapy will harm me a lot" can become "Chemotherapy helps me heal from cancer." You are not trying to cast the future in stone. You are trying to ease your mind and relieve fear, pain, and worry. Affirmations are possible in response to any and every concern. If I struggle with anxiety, I find an affirmation to be like an instant antidote to my fear.

WHAT ABOUT OPTIMISM?

At one point, early on in my cancer recovery, I realized that a lot of people were asking me to tell them my "prognosis." They were more or less subtle, depending on their personalities, but they did ask. When I said that I hoped to get better and not get cancer again, some of them were not satisfied. "But what are your chances?" Ugh. They wanted me to be realistic. Finally, one day, it popped out of my mouth: "Realism is over-rated, you know. I prefer to be optimistic. It's a lot easier." Why would I want to vote against myself or my chances of recovery?

When you resist optimism, you can feel burdened and discouraged. When you embrace optimism, you can take some steps towards recovering your health, however small those steps might seem. If you feel totally resistant to optimism, then you may want to discuss it with a spiritual person whom you trust, such as a counselor, pastor, or friend. You may want to read more about it. *Choosing To Be Happy* by Rick Foster and Greg Hicks is one of my favorite books, with its excellent research and lovely presentation style. *Flourish* is a new book by the champion of science-based optimism, Martin Seligman.

COPING WITH TROUBLESOME EMOTIONS

You won't exercise at all if you can't get out of bed because of your burden of depressive symptoms, so I am going to briefly address the issues of anxiety, fear, suffering, grief, and depression. Please get professional help if you need it. Keep in mind that exercise is very effective for treating mild depression. When you're stressed or blue, you have an ideal opportunity to use being physically active to help your spirits.

Seek Support and Community

If you are wrestling with cancer or cancer recovery, you are likely to face a full range of emotions and thoughts. First of all, try not to go through cancer recovery in isolation. Think beyond just your family and friends, if you need to. There are so many ways to find community support. Use resources at your hospital and in your community to find helpful support from groups or individuals.

Some fears are allayed quickly and easily when someone else says, "me, too." Cancer survivors share much in common with each other. It's as if we all speak the same foreign language about the disease. We all know cancer so well. It can be comforting just to realize that others have resolved through their fears, and you can too.

Acknowledge Emotions, Then Address Them

Patients who are always cheerful in the face of cancer, studies show, do not fare as well as those who express a variety of emotions. That's a reason to have at least one person to whom you are telling your truth. Your best choice is to acknowledge your actual fears, worries, and pains, then try to do something positive in reaction to them. The scariest emotions can be met with grace, empathy, love, and acceptance. In my experience, they then loosen their hold on me when I find a way to address my reality. Experiencing cancer is frightening, stressful, and often painful. To try to deny those things takes an enormous mental effort. Emotions, to me, are realities, first. Second, they are messages that we can use. Accepting how we feel, we know what to do next so that we can feel better. Use the messages the best ways that you can. If we first acknowledge how we feel, then we can try to soothe our fears, calm our minds, ease our pain and reduce our stress.

Perhaps you will want to explore more on this subject. Lawrence LeShan's *Cancer, A Turning Point*, is a classic book and its ideas are beautifully expressed. *Now That I Have Cancer, I Am Whole* is also a wonderful book written by John Robert McFarland, a minister who had cancer. For a discussion of health as it relates to how we live and what we believe, read *Choosing Health*, which is by the same authors as a *How We Choose to Be Happy*.

USING HEALING VISUALIZATIONS

One formal way to harness the positive power of your mind is to do a healing visualization, with guidance from a professional counselor or from an audiotape. Although the details vary, most approaches rely on the following three simple steps.

1. Evoke a state of relaxation so as to let the unconscious mind be receptive to positive imagery and affirmations. This is usually done by helping you to quiet the mind and it is similar to what is done with hypnosis, such as counting backwards slowly or focusing on a peaceful image.

2. Guide you to scan your body for tension and release it; to release fears and replace them with peaceful images; or to otherwise develop positive imagery to advance your healing.

3. The visualization will end with a sort of reverse of the initial process, thereby bringing you back to an ordinary state of mind, slowly and safely.

Some approaches use the model of the chakras or other specific healing models, but you should be able to find a guided visualization tape to suit your beliefs. A variety of CDs can be found in the Sounds True catalog of offerings on the Internet or in stores. I refer to two recordings in the resources section. The subconscious mind can help your immune system and advance your healing. The power of your mind is a great resource. Use it well.

BREATHING WELL WITH CONSCIOUS INTENTION

You are always breathing, but you are not always consciously aware of your breathing pattern. One great thing about aerobic exercise is that you can become more aware of your breathing. You can learn to breathe deeply and rhythmically during aerobic efforts by using your diaphragm to control your breath. A good way to practice your breathing is to breathe consciously while at rest.

Your diaphragm separates your lung cavity from your abdominal cavity. Here is a way to practice using your diaphragm muscle optimally. Assume a comfortable position sitting or lying down. Place your hand on your abdomen covering your navel with it. Take a deep breath in. Did your hand move towards your body or away from it? With the ideal breathing, your hand should move away from your body on the inhalation.

Chances are if you are untrained in belly breathing, your hand moved towards your spine as you breathed in. You probably took a deep breath by contracting your diaphragm muscle, which is the opposite of what you want to do. That movement actually makes the compartment containing your lungs smaller, not bigger.

To make your chest cavity bigger and give your lungs room to inflate to the best of their ability, you need to relax your diaphragm instead of contract it. Let's try again. On the in-breath, try to push out your abdomen and push your hand that is on your navel away from your spine. Feel it? Try again. Good.

If you have trouble, try starting with the out-breath during which you pull your belly inwards. That should allow you to relax your diaphragm on the in-breath that follows.

Here is another valuable breathing technique that you can use for relaxation. Read through these instructions and then try this exercise with your eyes closed.

Take a belly breath in by relaxing your diaphragm and expanding your lung space. For a moment, hold that breath in by simply being passive and not yet breathing out. Breathe out fully and deeply. Pause again, for a moment. Repeat this for five breaths.

Feel the difference? Presumably your heart rate lowered, your blood pressure lowered, your breathing rate reduced, your muscles generally relaxed, and your metabolism slowed. Not an unpleasant combination of effects.

Taking the time to pause between in-breaths and out-breaths helps your breathing to slow, but in also gives you conscious control of your breathing. This action is soothing. For more effect, try combining a simple word with your in-breath and another word with your out-breath.

I like to use this word combination: I breathe in while thinking of the word "love" and I breathe out "fear." I use those words because I often breathe with conscious intention when I am anxious. I like the image of expelling that which I want less. You may be able to identify two words that work best for you. Some people breathe in "peace" or "om." Some people choose a phrase with more words, such as "Calming my body, I breathe in. Caring for my body, I breathe out."

The simple process of paying attention to our breathing can be very relaxing and healing. You can do a breathing exercise for several breaths or for as long a time as you want to. Even 5 minutes of breathing slowly and deliberately is a very mean-ingful amount of time. Doing this exercise once or twice a day can really help your peacefulness, overall, and help you feel centered and relaxed.

You can also pay attention to your breath for several breaths while in the middle of other things like stressful phone calls, waiting on hold on the phone, talking to your doctor, or when you feel nervous for any reason. You can combine belly breathing or breathing intentionally with walking, running, or other activi-ties, as well. In fact, one of the reasons that exercise is relaxing is that it often involves breathing deeply. You can learn to enjoy breathing deeply, being relaxed, and feeling calm.

YOGA, CHI GONG, AND TAI CHI

Yoga has become accessible to most of us in yoga studios all across the country. Yoga classes are diverse in style and participants. Shop around until you find the class that suits you. Enjoy the experiential learning. Your yoga practice can be more than a convenient route to better flexibility and movement. If you are willing to explore yoga deeply with the right teachers, you will find many subtle benefits.

After a cancer diagnosis, many people will be open to changing their relationship with the idea of what it means to be alive, in this body, in this lifetime. Simply by calming the mind and making you feel present in your body, a yoga practice can be a holistic experience that speaks to your needs. I offer you encouragement to explore yoga for its subtle benefits, for its health effects, and for its holistic mind-body unity.

In addition to yoga, you may want to explore Chi Gong or Tai Chi. These two different, yet similar, Chinese arts involve gentle slow movements that are passed on from generation to generation. My experiences with Chi Gong and Tai Chi are extremely positive. I enjoy the flowing motions. After a short time doing the movements, I feel a greatly renewed sense of harmony within myself. Chi Gong, which has a history of medical use, can help your "energy" be balanced and help your health by regulating the flow of "Chi" or energy.

Tai Chi and Chi Gong practice may also be done in group classes in your community. These arts are ideal for people who do not have the strength for aerobic exercise but who crave some healing movement. One easy way to explore these two disciplines is to watch and learn through videos that you buy or find on YouTube. Gaiam has many DVDs of instruction. I like the DVDs by Linda Madoro very much.

※ ※ ※

ACTIVE SURVIVOR PROFILE: ELLEN

YOGA FOR HEALING, HELPING AND LIFE

Ellen Fein, currently a long-time survivor of acute myelogenous leukemia (AML), uses yoga, aerobic exercise activities, and strength training in her daily life. She walks outdoors in good weather for about 20 minutes each day. Ellen has some balance problems as a result of her cancer treatment side effects. In winter when ice and snow make sidewalks slippery, she goes to the gym to use the elliptical machine and recumbent bike. She also uses light free weights. Ellen isn't able to build much muscle mass or make many fitness gains because of some of her treatment side effects. Her exercise does help her to maintain her fitness to the degree that she can. She also feels that staying active helps her health in general.

Ellen's approach to her own healing is rooted in her daily yoga practice. Her morning begins with her yoga practice, which includes ritual, chanting and meditation as well as yoga poses and movement. In her yoga practice, as well as in daily living, she uses awareness of the breath and of yogic breathing techniques. Ellen says: "Movement is not the only avenue of healing." When she is not feeling well enough for movement, she emphasizes the other aspects of her yoga practice.

Prior to her cancer diagnosis, Ellen was very active in outdoor sports such as skiing, hiking, and biking. She also danced and did yoga. Her diagnosis of AML required intense treatment. She received her months-long chemotherapy in the hospital, during which time she was weak and nearly unable to stand up. After completing that treatment, she was able to recover some fitness. During the following year, however, Ellen needed stem cell transplantation, which has allowed her to achieve a lasting remission for the past ten years.

After completing the stem cell transplantation, Ellen rode her exercise bike and used free weights, despite weakness from side effects. She focused on breathing exercises and listened to music for relaxation during insomnia. She has chronic side effects, such as "exercise fatigue," which causes her muscles to stop working correctly after a relatively short period of time. She also has ongoing breathing problems and neurological problems, including difficulties with proprioception and balance. Her immune system "never completely reconstituted itself" and the donated stem cells that are now in her body tend to attack her own cells; medication, again with side effects, helps to control this.

Despite what to many people would be an inestimable health burden, Ellen has a calm and centered presence. In her community, Ellen shares her expertise and advocacy for holistic healing in a variety of ways. She is a licensed clinical social worker and a former staff member of a local oncology practice, where she provided coaching to patients who had cancer. She was able to bring tools such as guided visualization, breathing exercises, and the use of relaxation audio CDs to patients receiving chemotherapy. Ellen is currently self-employed as a "Cancer Coach" and a certified yoga therapist, helping people with cancer or chronic illnesses to establish tailored yoga practices to meet their individual needs.

Ellen authored a book, Not Just a Patient, and maintains a website of the same name. Her goals are "providing resources to assist individuals with chronic and life-threatening illness to develop a sense of well-being and to create quality in the life they have now." She established Michael's Fund in memory of her husband who passed away from cancer. The fund works to improve the conditions of people living with cancer in her region in association with a regional home health and hospice. Ellen also established a peer support network for cancer patients and produced a CD of healing visualizations.

"The idea is that we can all be active in our own healing," Ellen says. She sees the medical system, generally, as often ignoring the role that people can play in their own healing. She believes that the medical system focuses, for example, on using medications to solve problems with such things as anxiety, insomnia, and other normal human reactions to the stresses of a cancer ordeal. "I think that we can help people to be better at self-soothing," she said. Through her work with others, Ellen is, in her myriad ways, helping others to be more active in their own healing, just as she has been active in her own.

CHAPTER THIRTEEN

BE ACTIVE IN THE CANCER SURVIVOR COMMUNITY

Do you yearn to make a difference in the cancer community? There are a lot of ways that you can give to the cancer community by participating in athletic events that support cancer organizations. You can join with cancer survivors or others who support a good cause by participating in a race, a walk, or another activity that benefits a cancer-related organization. You can walk, run, bike, or snowshoe to raise money for cancer research. You can probably find something that suits you, close to home, or if not, you can network online and start your own event.

In the midst of hundreds or thousands of other cancer survivors, you can see how cancer reaches into many lives. You can see that you are far from alone with your disease. Meeting with healthy survivors, you may be inspired on your own healing path. You can help raise money, which feels good, and you can come home with new friends, a t-shirt, and a renewed sense of hope. There are so many ways to benefit by participating: it's a win-win situation, for you and the organization you support.

It would be quite impossible to catalog all of the cancer-related sports events. To find them, you only need to look around. I will describe a number of national programs, but you may also find local programs through your hospital, hospice, or United Way.

Because the cancer survivor community is large and diverse, you can probably find a place in it for yourself. The rather astonishing thing about the cancer survivor club, generally, is that once you are in the club, you're in. You have paid your dues by having a cancer diagnosis, and for the most part, you will find that the other club members can relate to your experiences. Although having had cancer is undesirable, you can eventually enjoy the camaraderie, empathy, and company of other cancer survivors.

WEAR YOUR SURVIVORSHIP ON YOUR SLEEVE

As an alternative to cancer-specific events, you can participate in any community run, bike ride, or other event while wearing a Livestrong bracelet, hat, shirt or something else that makes you feel proud to be a cancer survivor. Some of you may wear pink ribbons, Team-in-Training t-shirts, or other regalia. "Cancer sucks" t-shirts have their own brand appeal. Whatever you want your survivorship badge to look like, remember you are bringing awareness to cancer survivors everywhere. I find that my Livestrong hat or t-shirt makes me feel like I am being a good cancer survivor role model.

WHY BE PUBLIC ABOUT CANCER SURVIVORSHIP?

I heard Lance Armstrong speak at a cancer research fundraiser hosted by the Mary Haas Ovarian Cancer Early Detection Foundation in the fall of 2010. I have never felt as proud to be a cancer survivor as I felt when I was in the same room with the world-wide super-fighter of cancer, Lance Armstrong. Lance is the seven-time winner of the Tour de France, but he is more than a champion athlete. No one has changed the face of cancer survivorship more than he has with the combination of his remarkable cancer recovery, his athletic feats, and his worldwide fight against cancer.

Lance has helped cancer survivors to envision returning to great health after their harrowing cancer ordeals. When I was in chemotherapy, bald and fatigued, I was motivated by visions of Lance Armstrong pushing himself to the podium of the Tour de France. Just knowing that he had once battled cancer in the deep, dark trenches of a poor prognosis helped me realize that I could rise up from chemo-land to be fit again, even if not world-class fit. Looking at my Livestrong bracelet made me feel associated with the power and determination of cancer survivors around the globe.

Lance spoke about some advice that he received when he exited cancer treatment. His doctor told him he could leave through one of two doors: either the private door or the public door. If he went through the private door, he could just bury his cancer experience in the past and move on with his life. Or he could leave through the public door and take his cancer experience into the rest of his life. He could seek to give back to the cancer community. He could, as his doctor called it, respect the "obligation of the cured."

With Livestrong and its global campaign against cancer, Lance has excelled in the role of someone who took the public door. He makes it easier for any of the rest of us to do the same thing. Whether you want a yellow wristband yourself or not, whether you ever ride a bike or not, Lance Armstrong has changed how the world looks at cancer survivorship. I'm a fan of that effort.

I'm also a fan of the unknown thousands and thousands of cancer survivors who do a 5-kilometer walk, a 3-kilometer snowshoe, their first marathon or a lap around a track for cancer fundraising. Let's meet some of the organizations that make cancer advocacy their goal. If you choose to donate, make sure that you are comfortable with the allocation of your donations and the organization's overall financial priorities.

TEAM IN TRAINING

The brilliance of Team in Training (TNT) is four-fold. First, the organization takes individual sports, such as running, triathlon or biking, and makes them team sports by helping people train together. Second, qualified participating coaches and mentors help non-endurance athletes train to compete in endurance events, which can be life-changing and satisfying. Third, TNT raises money for blood cancer research for the Leukemia and Lymphoma Society. Lastly, the organization encourages cancer survivors to become lifelong athletes with group support, race experience and a positive attitude.

I have no experience with TNT myself, but I admire what they do. In the profile of endurance runner Newton Baker, you will learn about someone who has participated in TNT's group runs, gaining friends who share a blood cancer diagnosis. Betsy, another profiled survivor, trained to run her first marathon with TNT, waiting until after her race event to let her teammates know that she was a blood cancer survivor herself. There are so many different ways to get support and the quiet way worked for her.

What I admire most about TNT is that they take the illusion of competitiveness out of endurance racing. Let's face facts. So few participants line up at a marathon race with anything like a real chance of winning. That means most people are there for reasons other than strictly competing with each other. Team in Training puts the emphasis on team and training: I think that is brilliant—for cancer survivors or for anyone else. TNT also helps many non-endurance athletes learn to succeed at endurance sports. Success is all about the training. Do the training and you can succeed… and raise money for cancer research and make cancer-survivor friends.

LIVESTRONG

With about seven million yellow bracelets circling wrists all over the globe, the Livestrong Foundation, with its simple message of "live strong" has reached almost everyone. I love the name. Indeed, a cancer survivor can easily relate to wanting to live strong. What about beyond the message of living strong? What about the organization's activities and programs?

Livestrong produces fundraising athletic events, from bike rides to running races. Their Livestrong Challenges are races, in which participants raise money for the foundation from their friends and family members. Much like other athletic cancer-related, fundraising events, these events rely on participants' enthusiasm and their focused energy.

Livestrong has other components to its programs that may be less well known than the bracelets and the fundraising events. First, they have a cancer support line where you can receive guidance about coping with cancer and address issues of cancer survivorship. It's an amazing resource and it continues to grow.

Second, Livestrong has funded programs for cancer survivors at YMCAs across the country, in which they help cancer survivors achieve good levels of fitness for free or very inexpensively. See their website for a listing of current programs and contacts. These programs and other Livestrong initiatives have helped raise the bar for other cancer survivorship programs at hospitals and cancer centers.

Livestrong, in fact, has a special mission of improving the long-term medical care of cancer survivors, generally. They campaign on behalf of survivors' many needs, including areas of care that were previously underserved. If you have issues that extend past your active cancer treatment phase, sometimes it is hard to get medical help. Livestrong has modeled its survivorship care standards at pilot programs. It appears, to me, that their campaign for survivorship care has built significant momentum.

You should know that www.livestrong.com is not the right website address of the charitable foundation. Look at www.livestrong.org for the foundation's website. The dot-com is now run by a different for-profit company. The Livestrong Foundation continues to run as a non-profit organization with a board of directors and the structure of a charitable organization. The

Livestrong Foundation sponsors a cycling team, and Lance rode on the team with a yellow bracelet on his wrist to bring worldwide attention to Livestrong and cancer advocacy. Livestrong has recently passed the figure of 400 million dollars raised.

AMERICAN CANCER SOCIETY'S RELAY FOR LIFE

American Cancer Society's Relay for Life program is widespread and well established. It is also very successful at fundraising for the American Cancer Society. The ACS supports cancer research, programs for cancer survivors, and their Hope Lodges. These lodges, in various locations near hospitals, house cancer patients and caregivers receiving treatment far from their homes or for extended time periods.

The Relay-for-Life events have a format that includes teams that fundraise together and perform an all-night relay of walking around a track. Their motto is "cancer never sleeps." In that vein, the team members support each other in a night filled with music, special themes, and memorializing people by lighting candles in their honor. The American Cancer Society also uses the phrase: "Celebrate. Remember. Fight Back." In working together to get through the night's relay, team members may find solace, courage, and companionship.

The only on-snow relay is held at Trapp Family Lodge's esteemed cross-country ski center in Stowe, Vermont. I participated in this event less than one year after my cancer diagnosis. Being able to wear a survivor's sash and ski the opening lap with my husband wearing his caregiver's sash: quite an uplifting time. (It was there, amusingly, that my husband learned that "caregiver" was not a term that I had made up just for him. "I get a sash, too? You mean I have status?" he said.) Particularly touching to me were the paper lanterns with candles and messages about those who were lost to cancer.

I also enjoyed fundraising for the event. It was my first experience fundraising for a cancer organization. I wasn't sure what to expect, but it was easy. My friends and family responded positively to solicitations. I received some heartfelt messages of congratulations on my recovery. It was gratifying to see some good come from my cancer experience. Online tools made the process painless, logistically.

If you are at all team-oriented, you will like the Relay for Life's team focus. I haven't experienced a track-based walking Relay for Life, but those American Cancer Society events are very popular and successful. If you want to try fundraising in that atmosphere, look for an event near you.

SUSAN G. KOMEN RACE FOR THE CURE

Susan G. Komen was a successful woman who succumbed to breast cancer. She charged her sister with raising money to fight this horrible disease, and raise money, she has. The very successful Susan G. Komen Foundation is well known and nearly synonymous with the color pink, which they highlight in their various fundraising strategies. The foundation also sponsors the Susan Komen Race for the Cure in various locations across the country. The events, which once were woman-only, include cancer survivors, supporters and others. They present educational workshops and talks, along with the atmosphere of a large footrace, which includes several distances and welcomes walkers and runners alike.

ROMP TO STOMP OUT BREAST CANCER

A series of events in North America brings the sport of snow-shoeing to cancer fundraising. Begun in 2003 by the Tubbs snowshoe company, and currently run by Tubbs' new owner, the K2 ski company, the Romp to Stomp serves as an introduction to snowshoeing for about 25 percent of the participants. The thousands of snowshoers at nine different venues fundraise only if they want to, but fundraise they do, with a projected goal of $350,000 for 2011.

The family-friendly events feature both a snowshoe race and a snowshoe walk with the majority of people doing the walk. Tubbs snowshoes are provided for use, free of charge, at the events. New for 2011, a short course for children will be included, along with kids' separate registration pricing. Each cancer survivor gets a small gift—and a hug—at the Survivors' Tribute.

The well-run events also rely heavily on volunteer contributions, coordinated by one full-time K2 program administrator. Kristen, profiled in this book, tells of her successful multi-year participation and what it has meant to her. The program is a great way for people to exercise outdoors in winter with the support of other cancer survivors, while raising money for cancer research.

PULLING TOGETHER: THE DRAGON BOAT TEAM

Each summer, on Lake Champlain in Vermont, there is a Dragon Boat Festival. Originating in China, a dragon boat is a long narrow boat, propelled by about twenty paddlers. In the Dragonheart Vermont boat, women who are breast cancer survivors hold and use the single oars as they pull together. There is also a team leader onboard, functioning much like a coxswain by keeping the rhythm and shouting instructions. One participant told me about the dragon boat experience in these words: "The beauty of it is that you have to work together."

The paddling develops upper body strength, which can be helpful to breast cancer survivors. The team strives to create a sisterhood of breast cancer survivors, according to its brochure. The team practices together weekly in season, and travels to festivals monthly. Powering a boat together can bond the women to each other, make cancer's difficulties easier to face, and help with their health and well-being. Look for a dragon boat team near you.

Dragonheart Vermont has been so successful with their fundraising from their annual race event that they are in the middle of an initiative to offer survivorship care services to a broad range of cancer survivors. Their Survivorship Now program is an example of how the community of cancer survivors can benefit from local-based fundraising.

OTHER OPTIONS

Not every cancer type has its own fundraising sporting event. If you find yourself with a less common cancer, you still have various options. You can align yourself with the American Cancer Society, Livestrong, or other organization that is not specific to a certain type of cancer. You can see the whole of the cancer community as connected.

Perhaps you can find a less heralded cancer organization locally, such as at your local hospital, hospice or medical research center. Many places already have modest (or robust) fundraisers and they always need more volunteers. A regional hospital near me has had success with a group bike ride that raises large amounts of money for the cancer center. (See the Prouty Ride at www.dhmc.org.) Another popular format is a golf fundraiser. The Dana-Farber Cancer Center, in the Boston area, has its well-known Jimmy Fund whose events include nights at Fenway Park and the Pan-Mass Challenge, a bike ride. You can also find fundraising dances, if you would rather tap your heels than you tap your bike pedals. If your area is lacking fundraising events, why not start one that you would enjoy? Or, if you're not the organizing type, raise money with your own efforts by soliciting donations for your daily walks. For example, ask your friends if they would pledge a dollar a day for every day that you walked in a month. Be innovative. If you are sincere and trustworthy, it can all work out well.

The benefit of the formal fundraising events is that you are plugged in to a system that makes donors comfortable with secure online giving. If you do your own fundraising, you might have to restrict yourself to asking for money from people that you know well.

You may want to advocate for your fitness club to have a special workout class for survivors. You could start a yoga class for survivors in your community. You can start a weekly run or bike ride for survivors just for fun, community, and support. Please let your imagine run wild and then take some steps to help other cancer survivors be active and exercise.

Please also remember the cancer patients who are in hospice. Perhaps you can work with your hospice organization, locally, to bring some sort of movement therapy to hospice patients. Even if it is too late for a recovery, exercise such as gentle yoga can bring some happiness and distraction from pain.

Whatever you do, remember that you can make a meaningful difference in the cancer community by being as active and healthy as you can be. I hope that you enjoy exercising for your health all during your cancer recovery and beyond.

❀ ❀ ❀

ACTIVE SURVIVOR PROFILE: NEWTON

RUNNING TO HEALTH

When Newton Baker learned from his doctor that he had chronic lymphocyte leukemia, he listened to the doctor describe the disease. Then, Newton asked the doctor a critical question: "Can I keep running?"

Newton liked the answer. "Yes," his doctor said, "Exercise is the best thing that you can do for yourself. It will help your general health, it will help you build more red blood cells, and it will keep you happy."

That conversation took place nine years ago, and although Newton has the disease, he has not yet needed any medical treatment. The cancer is smoldering but has not progressed or caused any symptoms. And it has not caused Newton to stop running. Very little can stop Newton from running.

The day that I spoke with Newton Baker, age sixty-nine, he had just filled out some race entry forms for the following May. He'll do three half-marathons and two marathons that month. This kind of schedule is typical for him. He has competed in 139 marathons so far. And that's not even where Newton's agenda gets most interesting.

Newton has competed in the 24-hour running race format 23 times. In such races, you run as far as you can over a 24-hour period. Last time that he did so, he won his age group by running 90.9 miles. He stopped 80 minutes earlier than the 24-hour mark because he was a "little tired." He's not joking when he says this; Newton listens closely to his body's fatigue signals. He is able to do the high mileage that he does because he doesn't punish his body with pushing for his maximum speed all the time. With or without cancer, Newton is a poster boy of a remarkable, sensible, durable, if eccentric, endurance runner.

I have run with Newton in a local running club, so I was already familiar with his main tenet of his running philosophy: "Do not run to destruction." Newton believes that most runners who compete in races believe that they must run the most punishing pace that they can. He doesn't believe that approach is right. After copious research into running lore, including studying information on Navajo runners, the Wobblies in the 1800s, the Tamara Humara Indians, and other great runners, Newton decided that what makes a human animal able to run far and long is to run more slowly and to rest (or walk) when necessary.

For example, when he attempts the 24-hour run, he now aims for a 12-minute-per-mile pace. He trains more often at a 10-minute per mile pace. He has had to slow to compensate somewhat for his age. (No, he's not kidding.) By running at the 12-minute pace during 24-hour competitions, and by taking some nutrition every 4 miles, Newton is able to keep a pretty steady pace for the full 24 hours. Remarkable. (I honestly can't get my mind around this yet!)

Chronic lymphocytic leukemia isn't the only cancer he has faced. About three years ago, he learned that he had prostate cancer and needed a tiny malignant tumor removed. The surgery went well. And just under three weeks later, Newton ran a marathon in 4:32. He tosses in this disclaimer: "Well, I had been in pretty good shape before the surgery, having run two 24-hour events in the previous two months."

Newton runs based on how he feels. He wants to avoid pain or weakening his immune system. He quizzes his doctor about running and is reassured. "Whatever you are doing is working. Continue to do what you do. If you get sick or need treatment, we will make adjustments."

So far, so good. Perhaps one day, doctors will study Newton to see how what he does that keeps him healthy despite a blood cancer. Until then, you can keep in mind Newton's adage: "Don't run to destruction." You'll be likely to benefit your health long-term from slowing down your pace. It seems to be working out pretty well for him.

❄ ❄ ❄

ACTIVE SURVIVOR PROFILE: HELENE

RUNNING AWAY FROM CANCER: FAR AWAY

Helene Neville knows two kinds of pain: the kind that has been forced upon her by cancer, surgery, radiation and related suffering and the kind that she has chosen to impose on herself through running. She calls the latter type of pain "good pain." When Helene's medical caregivers told her in 1998 that she should "get her affairs in order," after brain cancer treatment options were exhausted, Helene accepted their verdict. However, she didn't accept the idea that she should just wait for the disease to win. Helene thought she might as well have "good pain" on her own terms and create some positive memories for her family. Facing a terminal prognosis, Helene started to get ready to run a marathon.

However, most people would not call running a few times adequate preparation for a marathon. Helene's longest run was six miles, but that preparation was all she could manage. She was too sick and too weak to run more. Ready or not, Helene ran her first marathon in 1998, in Chicago. A former track runner, she finished in a respectable 4 hours and 28 minutes. This race result led her to wonder if she was a natural endurance runner. (Answer: yes.) Certainly, she was mentally tough. Not giving up on life seemed to be working for her.

Helene relates that her doctors were neutral about exercise at the time, but when she turned to running, she seemed to run away from cancer. Far away–all the way back to health. Helene went on to compete in many marathons, become a winning body-builder, and live cancer-free. Clearly, the doctors had underestimated her ability to recover. Her survival was exceptional. And Helene did more than survive: she thrived.

Twelve years later, in 2010, Helene was the picture of health as she finished another notable long-distance event. She ran across the United States from the Pacific Ocean to the Atlantic Ocean in 93 days. She averaged about 50 miles each day, by doing 10-minute miles and sustaining a phenomenal pace over such a distance.

Helene, a long-time nurse, has also authored a book, Nurses in Shape, in which she conveys her hope that the nursing professionals can improve their own health in order to be better role models themselves. Helene is a model of determination, hope, and steady pace. She thinks that exercise is a big boost to her health, and she is glad that "exercise is free." Anyone can do it. She advises starting with small goals and building up from there. Helene pays a lot of attention to nutritional choices. She has embraced a holistic approach to eating as put forth at the Oasis Center of Healing in Mesa, Arizona.

Helene is an awesome advocate for others staying healthy with exercise. She has already beaten the odds. She likes her chances of being healthy for a long time to come. Interestingly, she's planning another cross-country run for 2011, this time from Canada to Mexico. Check out her website, www.oneontherun.com, and maybe you can show her some cancer survivor support along the way.

AFTER CANCER, MY FIRST RACE BACK

I have been lucky. In the four years since my cancer diagnosis, I have stayed healthy. In general, since cancer, I have been able to do my sports, rejoin competition, and enjoy the blessing of having no evidence of disease. I have skied in a 25-km race, run a half-marathon race, and treasured many great outings to swim, run or hike. Some days, I can see my cancer ordeal as something in the past and my memories of it are starting to dim. I do remember certain milestones, of course. I would like to share this final memory with you.

About one month after treatment, I went down to a spot a few miles from my house and watched hundreds of runners in a half-marathon running race go by. I was sitting in the sun, with my Livestrong yellow cap over my still bald head.

The race was special to me. It was run on the same half-marathon course that was my first half-marathon ever, in 1993. The year that I finished chemo, many of my friends from my old running club were running in it. I saw one friend, Anne, coming towards me as she raced. I had shared many companionable miles with her over the years. I said hello from my spot on the sidelines.

Anne did a double-take when she recognized me. One second later, she looked like she was going to cry, seeing me sitting there, looking just like a post-chemo cancer survivor. I tried to smile and convey that I was okay. She didn't look convinced, but I was at peace with myself. Treatment was over, and I was pretty confident that my health would return. I promised myself I would be running that race the following year.

Fast-forward one year. The same annual half-marathon race was on my agenda. I wasn't well prepared, but I was going to run it anyway. Honestly, I was poorly prepared. Instead of training properly, I had been making frequent 100-mile car trips to help with my dad's hospice care. He was dying of cancer at his home. I was going to run the half-marathon as a tribute to his fighting spirit, as much as in celebration of my own health. I knew I could run the distance on my background of fitness and the fuel of my grief.

My father was tough: the cancer that was beating him was his fourth type of cancer. He claimed that he had always been lucky, and he said that it just made sense that he would run out of luck at some point. He wasn't going to complain at this juncture, he said. A pragmatic—or was it philosophical—retired physician, he was eighty-four. At the time of my race, he was in his third month of being bed-ridden at home, cared for by my mother and others. I didn't really have the words for my grief, but the long race-course offered me a kind of symbolic time to imagine saying goodbye to him. He passed away four weeks later.

During the warm-up, before the race, I saw quite a few friends, including my friend Anne. I was met with a big hug, and again she appeared emotionally moved. There was happiness in her eyes, though. I could see that this year she was relieved to see me with a race bib announcing that I was running the full distance. The only way I looked like a cancer survivor was that my hair was still short with its trademark post-chemo curls. Anne was happy to see me lacing up my shoes.

The first half of the race went great, then my lack of preparatory miles caught up with me. I slowed down and my feet, never one hundred percent since their experience of peripheral neuropathy, started to hurt with each step. In later miles, I tried to walk, but the pain on my soles was crippling at the slow speed. I ran slowly and finished well back in the pack. I suffered with each footfall in those last five miles, but I kept thinking, "This is for you, Dad." I knew his suffering was worse than my own.

When I crossed the finish line, I was as proud as ever in racing. I felt less like a cancer patient and more like a cancer survivor. I felt that I was putting some distance between my life and my cancer, even though I was also sad about my father's cancer. I had made some peace with what was going on in my life.

In a strange twist, the race left me with a special prize. My feet used to hurt every time I ran post-chemotherapy; since that race, they have never hurt again. I had wondered, in the late miles of that race, if I was ruining my feet. Instead, the peripheral neuropathy seemed cured by that race. I don't understand it, but I'll take it. I am lucky.

I hope that you can one day look over your shoulder while you walk, run, or ride, and see cancer back there, way behind you, winded, bent over and quitting while you stride onward.

I wish you well.

Your friend,
Nancy S. Brennan

Sources Cited
and Further Resources

SOURCES CITED

American Cancer Society. *www.americancancersociety.com.* July 1, 2010.

Cochrane Review. *Cochrane Library,* No. 6, 2010.

American College of Sports Medicine. *www.acsm.org.* Article: "ACSM / ACS Certified Exercise Trainer", accessed January 2011.

Armstrong, Lance. *It's Not About the Bike: My Journey Back to Life.* Penquin Putnam Group, 2000.

Block, Keith I. *Life Over Cancer.* Bantam, Random House, 2009.

Block Center for Integrative Cancer Treatment, *www.blockmd.com,* accessed February 2011.

Cancer Center of Santa Barbara, *www.ccsb.org* for information on Well-fit program, accessed March 2011.

Cancer Treatment Centers of America, *www.cancercenter.com/ complementary-alternative-medicine/physical-therapy.cfm,* accessed March 2011.

Dartmouth-Hitchcock Medical Center, *Video on Exercise for Breast Cancer Patients.* with support of Vermont-New Hampshire Affiliate of the Susan G. Komen For the Cure and Dartmouth-Hitchcock Medical Center, Lebanon, New Hampshire. July 1, 2010. www.dhmc.org.

Dittus, Kim, M.D., Ph.D. "Exercise During and Beyond Breast Cancer Therapy." *2010 Breast Cancer Conference, Stowe, Vermont.* Seminar presentation.

Dreyer, Danny. *Chi Running: A Revolutionary Approach to Effortless, Injury-Free Running.* Fireside of Simon and Schuster, 2004.

Keane, Maureen and Daniela Chace, *What to Eat if You Have Cancer*. McGraw Hill Books, 1996.

Lerner, Michael, *Choices in Healing: Integratring the Best of Complementary and Conventional Approaches to Cancer*. MIT Press, 1994.

LeShan, Lawrence. *Cancer As a Turning Point: A Handbook for People with Cancer, Their Families, and Health Professionals*. Plume of Penquin/Putnam Group, 1990.

Litterini, Amy, *A Model Cancer Wellness Program: Exercise and Art in Cancer Survivorship*, www.accc-cancer.org/education/pdf/edu_CoSS_litterini.pdf, accessed March 2011

McFarland, John Robert. *Now That I Have Cancer I Am Whole*. Andrews-McMeel Publishing, 2007.

National Cancer Institute. "Fact Sheet on Physical Activity and Cancer." *National Cancer Institute*. July 1, 2010. www.cancer.gov.

Schmitz, Kathryn, Ph. D. et al. "American College of Sports Medicine Roundtable on Exercise Guidelines for Cancer Survivors." *Official Journal of American College of Sports Medicine*, June 1, 2010: 1409-1426.

Servan-Schreiber, David, M.D., Ph.D. *Anticancer, A New Way of Life*. Viking Penquin, Penquin Group, 2008.

Stinchfield, Kate. "Cancer: more exercise, not less, may be the best" *www.health.com*. June 12, 2010.

FURTHER RESOURCES: BOOKS, CDS AND DVDS

Anderson, Greg. *Cancer: 50 Essential Things To Do*. Plume, Penquin Group, 1999.

Arem, Kimba and Andrew Weil, M.D. *Self-healing with Music and Sound*, (CD). Sounds True, 2005.

Arnot, Robert. *The Biology of Success*. Little, Brown, 2000.

Baker, Dan, and Cameron Stauth. *What Happy People Know: How the New Science of Happiness Can Change Your Life for the Better*, St. Martin's Press, 2003.

Blaylock, Russell L. *Natural Strategies for Cancer Patients.* Twin Streams Health, Kensington Publishing Group, 2003.

Bourne, Edmund and Lorna Garano, *Coping with Anxiety.* New Harbinger, 2003.

Bray, Sharon. *When Words Heal: Writing Through Cancer.* Frog Limited c/o North Atlantic Books, 2006.

Bristow, Robert E and F.J. Montz. *A Guide to Survivorship for Women with Ovarian Cancer.* The Johns Hopkins University Press, 2005.

Browning, Ray and Rob Sleamaker. *Serious Training for Endurance Athletes.* Human Kinetics, 1996.

Carr, Kris. *Crazy Sexy Cancer Tips.* Skirt! 2007.

Chace, Daniella and Maureen Keane. *What to Eat if You Have Cancer: A Guide to Adding Nutritional Therapy to Your Treatment Plan.* McGraw Hill, 1996.

Dyer, Diana. *A Dietician's Cancer Story.* Swan Press, 1997.

Davies, Brenda. *The 7 Healing Chakras.* Ulysses Press, 2000.

Dadd, Debra Lynn. *Home Safe Home: Protecting Yourself and Your Family from Everyday Toxics and Harmful Household Products.* Jeremy P. Tarcher/Putnam of Penquin Putnam, 1997.

Douillard, John. *Body, Mind and Sport: The Mind-Body Guide to Lifelong Fitness and Your Personal Best.* Crown Trade Publishing, 1994.

Dyer, Diana. *A Dietician's Cancer Story.* Swan Press, 1997.

Foster, Rick and Greg Hicks. *Choosing Brilliant Health.* Penguin Group, 2008.

Gaemi, Sonia. *Eating Wisely for Hormonal Balance.* New Harbinger, 2004.

Huang, Chungliang Al and Jerry Lynch. *Working Out, Working Within*. Jeremy P. Tarcher/Putnam.

Haas, Elson M. *The Detox Diet*. Celestial Arts, 1996.

Hicks, Greg and Rick Foster. *Choosing Brilliant Health*. Penquin Books, 2008.

Lawson, Lynn. *Staying Well in a Toxic World: Understanding Environmental Illness, Mulitple Chemical Sensitivities, Chemical Injuries and Sick Building Syndrome*. Lynnword Press, 1993.

Modaro, Linda. *Discovering Chi: Energy Exercises for the Beginner* (DVD). Terra Entertainment, 2005.

Maffetone, Philip. *The Maffetone Method: The Holistic, Low-Stress No-Pain Way to Exceptional Fitness*. McGraw-Hill. 2000.

Martin, Chia. *Writing Your Way Through Cancer*. Hohm Press, 2000.

Murray, Michael, and Tim Birdsall, Joseph Pizzorno, Paul Reilly. *How to Prevent and Treat Cancer with Natural Medicine*. Berkeley Publishing Group, Penquin Group, 2002.

Millman, Dan. *Body Mind Mastery*. New World Library, 1999.

Mittleman, Stu. *Slow Burn: Burn Fat Faster by Exercising Slower*. Quill, Harper Collins, 2000.

Ojeda, Linda. *Menopause Without Medicine*. Hunter House, 2003.

Pizzorno, Joseph. *Total Wellness*. Prima Publishing, 1996.

Rossman, M.D., Martin, *Guided Imagery for Self-Healing*. New World Library/H J Kramer Book, 2000.

Sat Dharam Kaur, Mary Danylak-Arhanic, and Carolyn Dean. *The Complete Natural Medicine Guide to Women's Health*. Robert Rose, 2005.

Schwarz, Anna L. *Cancer Fitness*. Fireside, Simon and Schuster, 2004.

Seligman, Martin. *Flourish: A Visionary New Understanding of Happiness and Well-being*. Free Press, May 2011.

Siegel M.D., Bernie S. *Love, Medicine and Miracles*. Harper and Row, 1986.

Seigel M.D., Bernie S. *Meditations for Morning and Evening: Start Your Day with Confidence and Ease, Two Powerful and Original Guided Imagery Meditations*, (CD). Hay House, 2004.

Silver, Julie K. *After Cancer Treatment*. Johns Hopkins University Press, 2006.

Somers, Suzanne. *Knockout: Interviews with Doctors Who Are Curing Cancer and How to Prevent Getting It in the First Place."* Crown, 2009.

Stauth, Cameron and Dan Baker. *What Happy People Know*. St. Martin's Press, 2003.

Stockdale, Brenda. *You Can Beat the Odds*. Sentient , 2009.

Ryan, Monique. *Sports Nutrition for Endurance Athletes*. Velo Press, 2007.

Rossman, Martin L. *Guided Imagery for Self-Healing*. H. J. Kramer, 2000.

Viscott, David. *Emotional Resilience*. Three Rivers Press, 1996.

Weil M.D., Andrew, *Natural Health, Natural Medicine: A Comprehensive Manual for Wellness and Self-Care*. Houghton Mifflin, 1990.

Weil M.D., Andrew. *Spontaneous Healing*. Random House Publishing Group, 1995.

Weil, M.D., Andrew and Martin Rossman, M.D. *Self-healing with Guided Imagery*, (CD). Sounds True, 2003.

FURTHER RESOURCES: ON THE WEB

American Cancer Society, www.americancancersociety.org

Breast cancer information, www.breastcancer.org

Cancer Center of Santa Barbara, www.ccsb.org

Casting for Recovery, www.castingforrecovery.org

Donna Deegan's "Donna Foundation," www.thedonnafoundation.org

Dragonheart Vermont, www.dragonheartvermont.org

Ellen Fein, www.notjustapatient.com

Exeter Hospital, www.exeterhospital.com

Expedition Inspiration, www.expeditioninspiration.org

Gaiam for yoga and other instructional DVDs, www.gaiam.com

Helene Neville, www.oneontherun.com

Information on Livestrong's YMCA cancer survivor programs, www.livestrong.org

John Bigham, aka The Penguin, www.johnbigham.com

Moving On Aerobics, www.movingonaerobics.org

Prevention magazine, www.rodale.com

Romp to Stomp Out Breast Cancer, www.tubbsromptostomp.org

Sounds True Catalog, guided meditations and more, www.soundstrue.com

Susan G. Komen for the Cure, www.komen.org

Team-in-Training, www.teamintraining.org

Urbanzen Foundation for yoga therapy information, www.urbanzen.org

APPENDIX

EXERCISE IN BALANCE WITH HEALTHY EATING

With a cancer challenge comes an incentive to eat healthy foods. No matter how well or how poorly you have nourished yourself in the past, you can make a meaningful contribution to recovering your health through improved nutrition. Although complete nutritional guidance is beyond the scope of this book, I will make some suggestions based on reading, research with nutritionists, and personal experience.

I recommend that you also find your own trusted sources, be they a nutritionist, a book by Dr. Andrew Weil or another trusted expert, or a magazine like *Eating Well, Prevention,* or *Everyday Food.* Please also check with your physicians or a nutritionist who works with cancer patients for specific recommendations for your own health status. Here are some general guidelines.

- Do you need to lose body fat and gain muscle, maintain your weight, or gain weight to achieve a good body composition? Knowing what your goals are helps you think clearly about your food needs. Depending on your cancer and cancer treatment, any of these three options are possible. Discuss this openly with your doctor so you know which applies to you.

- Be aware that sometimes if you start at a pretty good body weight, doing more exercise and eating well can add some body weight because you lose fat but gain muscle. Don't focus on the number on the scale in such an instance: Focus on how you feel. If you are getting stronger and fitter, it's okay sometimes to gain pounds.

- Make the most of your meal times. Eat well at your meal times. Include ample fresh vegetables and fruits, whole grains, unprocessed foods, good fats like those in nuts or olive oil, and lean proteins. Eat proportional to your caloric needs for the day. A small amount of good fat consumed at each meal helps your body perform the best. Some protein consumed after exercise can help your muscles recover.

- If you are experiencing nausea or other challenges to feeling hungry, try to take in the right amount of calories for the day, anyway. If necessary, eat smaller meals; eat four or five times during the day. Get medical help and/or use safe home remedies for nausea, if it interferes greatly with your ability to eat well.

- Limit your intake of refined sugar to almost none. If you can keep your blood sugar level, you will have your best chance of naturally wanting to eat good foods. Eating refined sugars spikes your insulin level, which is not good for a cancer patient. Eating sugar also tends to create a pattern of eating poorly to satisfy cravings that happen when the blood sugar later drops.

- To best even out blood sugar, eat low on the glycemic index by eating foods that have complex, not simple, sugars. Such food digests more slowly, helping you feel better. For example, bread with whole grain and almond butter will leave you satisfied longer than a refined-flour sugar-laden cereal for breakfast. A brown rice and veggie salad will leave you satisfied longer than cake and cookies. Invest some time in familiarizing yourself with the glycemic index and what foods are best for keeping your blood sugar level.

- Drink plenty of water. Don't drink overly sweetened drinks often or at all. Squeeze a lemon into a glass of water for a quick refresher that is good for your liver's health. Use agave nectar or honey as a sweetener instead of white sugar. Drink green tea (check with your doctor) for its anticancer properties if appropriate to your situation.

- Eat mindfully, slowly and with enjoyment.

- Eat as many organically grown foods as possible. See the book, *Anticancer*, for more detail on the hazards of chemically laden foods.

- If you have had trouble with obesity or being badly overweight your whole life, seek appropriate professional help now. Why not address this now with adequate support?

- Exercise a small amount before each meal if you struggle with a low appetite. A 5-minute walk may stimulate your appetite enough to make you choose good foods.

- Make it simple to eat well by only buying good, healthy foods. Don't stock up on anything that you don't believe is good for you.

- If you are too run-down to prepare good foods for yourself, ask for help from friends who might bring you some good prepared food.

- Take a multivitamin, if your doctor approves. Also consider your vitamin D, calcium, and magnesium needs; your need for essential fatty acids; and, taking probiotics or eating yogurt.

OTHER HEALING MODALITIES

This book has focused on healing with exercise activities, but, as you know, there are many different integrative therapies that can be used in combination with standard medical approaches. Many physicians are open-minded about your judicious use of safe home remedies, acupuncture, and various supplements.

You will want to make sure that you keep your treating physician informed about anything that you are doing that could affect your treatment outcome along these lines. You want to be sure not to interfere with your treatment's effectiveness. For more information, the Mayo Clinic has a good resource online about possible contraindications to common supplements. Err on the side of caution.

Find multiple sources of reliable information and get your doctor's okay before trying anything. Specific recommendations are not appropriate to this book, but I will drop a few hints here. Take this advice as you would take it from any well-meaning cancer survivor whom you don't know.

Michael Lerner's esteemed book, *Choices in Healing*, used very strict standards to measure the research results of use of alternative healing modalities. Acupuncture was the most powerful choice, he found, in treating cancer patients. I strongly suggest that you pursue acupuncture with the best acupuncturist that you can find. I was lucky to have two wonderful acupuncturists help in my care and recovery.

Supplements, such as herbs and vitamins, need an entire book themselves. See the resources section for ideas. I looked into using mushroom extract, curcumin, melatonin, a multi-vitamin, essential fatty acids, and green tea. You will have your own ideas.

Lastly, do not underestimate the value of counseling by people who are trained to help with cancer issues. A support group or individualized counseling may be appropriate. Some diagnoses and treatments are capable of causing post-traumatic stress disorder, for which help should be available if you ask for it. Please do not suffer in isolation or without the help you need. Unconventional counseling with a person trained in ancient healing arts like Chi Gong or shamanism can be beneficial. Don't let anyone judge you for your choices.

Also, massage therapists sometimes receive training in lymph drainage, which can be useful in healing. Plus, many massage therapists are by nature compassionate and caring, as well as professional. They have many different types of massage that they can use, not just sports massage. You may enjoy the relaxation enormously during your stressful cancer challenge. Take good care of yourself.

INFORMATION ABOUT OVARIAN CANCER

For more information about ovarian cancer, please see these websites.

Eleanor B. Daniels Fund, www.ebdfund.org

Mary Haas Ovarian Cancer Early Detection Foundation, www.maryhaasfoundation.org or see their Facebook page

National Ovarian Cancer Coalition, www.ovarian.org

Ovarian Cancer National Alliance, www.ovariancancer.org

Web-MD website's ovarian cancer information: www.webmd.com/ovarian-cancer

For a listing of more websites: www.ovariancancer.jhmi.edu/resources.cfm

Four Signs of Ovarian Cancer:

- Bloating
- Pelvic or abdominal pain
- Difficulty eating or feeling full quickly
- Urinary symptoms (urgency or frequency)

Women who have these symptoms almost daily for more than a few weeks should see their doctor, preferably a gynecologist, according to press release in 2007 by national ovarian cancer organizations.

Ovarian cancer needs more champions. Here are two new organizations that are trying to make a difference—and succeeding.

Clearity Foundation

The Clearity Foundation is a relatively new organization advancing the testing of ovarian cancer tumors so that the "profiling" information can help inform the treatment choices and advance better treatments using molecular information to fit drug choices to the patient's tumor's genetic make-up. Please support this important initiative by see their website at www.clearityfoundation.org.

The Mary Haas Ovarian Cancer Early Detection Foundation

Founded after the death of Mary Haas from ovarian cancer, this foundation has a specific and important mission of helping advance the early detection of ovarian cancer. Early detection could save many lives because so many cases of ovarian cancer are detected at late stages. This young organization has already exhibited powerful fundraising abilities so look to its website for more information or to get involved.

ON THE SUMMIT IN SUMMER

©Nancy S. Brennan

I never dreamed that I would want
an oxygen tank on my back
so that I could walk up the hill
to my house. I never
dreamed of a lot of the things
that happen in chemotherapy,
humbling, painful, personal things,
but I dreamed of this moment: standing
on my favorite mountain summit
in mid-summer, bald, tired
and grinning like the blessed fool
that I am. I am
incredulous at the sight
of all that is living, all that life,
in the woods, hills and houses,
below and beyond. It's Vermont,
New York, Canada and New Hampshire
that I can see, not the Himalayas. This is
just Camel's Hump Mountain
and from this high rocky peak, I can see
my house, four miles west as the crow flies,
six miles away by foot. I came the last
three miles up the trail by foot
to where my soul likes best to be.
I can see past the foreground
Of my fear and suffering. I can see past
cancer all the way to the horizon
of ordinary life
where I aim to return when I have
enough stamina and strength—and
the doctors I'm okay.
Right now, it is enough to have glimpsed my
recovery. In the weird world
that they call cancer treatment, it is
enough to be taking small, slow steps
toward a landscape without disease.

About the Author

Outdoor athlete, writer, and health advocate, Nancy Smith Brennan lives in central Vermont with her family. She has worked as a natural resources planner, teacher, writer, editor, Nordic ski instructor, and farmhand. Nancy is also a poet. She holds a bachelor's degree from Middlebury College in Biology, with a minor in Creative Writing. This is her first book. She has a master's degree in Regional Planning from the University of Massachusetts at Amherst. She is an avid gardener, seamstress and birdwatcher.

You can find out more about this book, as well as the "Active Against Cancer" workshops, at www.activeagainstcancerbook.com.

Nancy Brennan owns Birdsbesafe LLC, which makes and sells the Birdsbesafe™ cat collar, which protects songbirds from the hunting of outdoor housecats. See www.birdsbesafe.com for more information.

Made in the USA
Lexington, KY
26 October 2011